PSYCHOLOGY OF DAILY HOLISTIC

YOGA

AND SELF REALIZATION

DR. LAUTURE MASSAC

Published Massac in USA

Second edition, 2018
10 9 8 7 6 5 4 3 2 1

Massac, Lauture.
Psychology of daily holistic yoga and self-realization: Lauture Massac.
ISBN 978-0-692-18188-1

1. Hatha yoga. 2. Kundalini. 3. Yoga, Kriya. 4. Yoga, Raja. 5. Yogis -
United States. 6. Yogis – India. 7. Meditation.

DISCLAIMER: The author of this book does not dispense medical
advice nor prescribe the use of any technique as a form of treatment for
medical problems without the advice of a physician. The intent of the
author is to offer information that is general in nature. The author and
publisher assume no responsibility for your actions in the event you use
the information in this book for yourself.

Printed and bound in the United States. The text paper is SFI certified. The Sustainable
Forestry Initiative® program promotes sustainable forest management.

DEDICATION

A special remembrance to my Guru brother Yogi Amrit Desai, one of the great pioneers of yoga in the West. When we met in 1971 in Rishikesh, India, his invitation to me to meet his guru, Bapuji Swami Shri Kripalu, has changed my life.

This book is also dedicated to all other pioneers of yoga in Western countries. To all gurus, Yoga instructors who have established yoga studios, centers, and ashrams, and by their good will, in one way or the other, have brought wellness, peace, and hope to millions.

INTRODUCTION

Since the appearance of man on earth, he has always felt the vulnerability of the body. Living under the sky and constantly experiencing the forces of nature, he is overcome by fears which create the need to seek for some protection.

He wishes to protect the body from injuries, diseases, and even death. He worships different things in nature his imagination may consider as a wonder, such as the sun, the moon, the rivers, some curious stones, trees, etc. In his search for body control, he discovers the secret virtue of many plants which cure diseases, give health, and even offer some psychedelic experiences.

It is written in the Bible the story of some men who could live several hundred years (Genesis 5.5; 5:27, 9:29). To live such a long life they must have had some deep secret knowledge of the body.

During the first Olympiad in 776 B.C., the games were practiced not only for entertainment, but also for good health and body control (Spivey, N. 2012). Therefore, it can be stated that humans have not been created to remain still like a tree. One feels the need to move the limbs, to curve the body up and down, and to turn. From this point of view, it can be stated that from the beginning of creation humans were unknowingly practicing a kind of yoga.

When you get up in the morning, your first reaction is to straighten out your legs and arms, to regulate automatically your breath, and to yawn. Is yoga the invention of any one person? Certainly not. It is virtually in everyone, including the animals. However, it is only in humans that yoga could be fully developed.

Even Vacaspati and Vijnana Bhiksu, the two great commentators on the Vyasabhasya, agree and in holding that Maharishi Patanjali, the well-known author of the Yoga Sutras, was not the creator of the yoga, but only an editor (Misra, V. 1974). Also, the analytic study of the sutras strengthens the conviction that the sutras do not show any original attempt, but a mastery and systematic compilation which was also supplemented by fitting contribution.

The systematic manner in which the first three chapters are written by way of definition and classification also shows that the materials were already in existence and that Patanjali only systematized them.

Many scholars have tried to settle a date for the appearance and origin of yoga, but they have failed. Maharishi Patanjali, who wrote the yoga sutras in about the year 200 B.C., was not the first author on the subject. It is known that much earlier some other rishis had written such Upanishads on yoga, including Sandilys, Yogattwa, Dhyanabindu, Hamsa, Amritanada, Varasha, Mandala, Brahmana, Nadabindu, and Yoga Kundalini Upanishads.

It can also be stated that the science of yoga is not the prerogative of India, though it seems that it originated there. There is a wrong belief in some people thinking that besides the workout form of yoga, which is practiced in many studios in the United States, Westerners are not fit for the practice of real esoteric yoga. Yoga should suit all human beings, no matter what country they belong to, because it is already in the body of everyone.

Medical science reveals that one of the main causes of heart attack is plaque build-up in the arteries, leading to poor blood circulation. Have you not seen a pipe in which clean water is not flowing properly for many months? What happens? It becomes congested and all kinds of bacteria have developed in it. The same phenomenon is happening in a human body in which the blood is not circulating properly. Infection begins to develop, and all kinds of diseases are ready to attack the organs. A dead body will decompose within a few hours because there is no blood circulation.

The yogic exercises will not only help the blood to circulate well in the veins, but they will purify them as well. Yoga is more than ordinary physical exercises practiced for body fitness. The yogic asanas, when performed slowly and in the right way, go deep into the cells of the body, purify the blood, and wash away hidden diseases.

What is the goal of life if it is not happiness? Then what else could it be? Everyone on earth wishes to be happy, which is the birthright of all of us. As a youngster, while living under the roof of our parents, we struggle to get an education and to develop the intellect in order to occupy a good position in society. A similar struggle is to succeed in business and to accumulate material wealth. Unfortunately, many people are sometimes seeking happiness in the wrong way. In wealthy societies, we often see many overweight children who become obese adults with all of the health consequences. The body, which is the vehicle in which all of these desires could be achieved, is usually neglected. The diseases therefore have signed a compromise with the body. They keep scourging it from time to time, and even if wealth and fame are achieved, there is not permanent joy or happiness. The mind and the body are not in harmony.

The goal of yoga through personal experience is to help one achieve good health with a balanced mind in a healthy body. When peace and joy are achieved within, then it becomes possible to spread happiness in our surroundings through divine love. Because of the suffering, it could be very difficult for a sick person to make his or her surrounding happy. Psychologically and emotionally, a sick person feels powerless, unconcerned with the notion of happiness, and becomes a source of constant worries for the loved ones. Yoga will help one achieve self-control, self-confidence, and a sound mind and body.

People who identify themselves with all the worldly advertisements they are receiving every day through technology, and who consider the body as a garbage bag into which everything goes, have to keep permanently in their medicine cabinet a private pharmacy. Their entire lives depend on medications. Whenever abnormality of blood pressure or blood sugar is disturbing the body, they have to rush to the medicine cabinet for some relief pills. For them, it is easier to swallow a pill and to feel temporarily better than to follow a yogic discipline which will bring a stable health condition. However, one thing to remember is that every time a drug is introduced into the body, it creates a negative reaction in different parts of the system.

The practice of regular yoga asanas keeps the body warm and purifies the blood. Circulation is better achieved in the arteries; the muscles and the joints will get relief from pain. A person suffering from rheumatoid arthritis will benefit greatly from regular gentle yoga postures. Many practitioners of hatha yoga who had symptoms of arthritis have reported great improvements in their lives, with decrease of inflammation and more joint flexibility.

There is an old saying that "most troubles are manmade." If a person is living an intelligent life, in harmony with nature and without abusing the body, that individual should usually enjoy a healthy life with no chronic disease. We can say that the body needs three basic things to stay healthy: pure air, proper food, and exercise.

For example, take a dog who is living in nature—he is full of energy. He gets enough space to run, to exercise his limbs, and to breathe fresh air. Such dog will probably die of old age without any disease. But take another dog which has been quite healthy in the wild. Now he is adopted and is living in an apartment. He is getting special dog food. Though he is living a comfortable life surrounded by the full loving care of his master and away from fear of possible attacks from predators, you will notice as years go by that he will develop the same type of diseases to which humans are victims (cancer, ulcers, arthritis, etc.). There is nothing as pure as natural living with plenty of fresh air and open space to move around.

Yes, yoga is a preventive as well as a curative science. However, one should not wait until the body is invaded with diseases to start practicing yoga, or to expect a curative miracle. The health-oriented person will take advantage of the youthful body to start the practice of yoga. If a young person was not aware of the benefits of yoga or did not have the opportunity to practice it, and now old age is showing, and aches and pains are attacking the body, yoga can still help. However, one should not expect a curative miracle. According to my teaching experience, many people with a worn-out body, which medical science cannot help anymore, come to yoga after suffering for many years and expect to get cured within ten days. If that expected miracle did not happen within that short period of time, they give up the practice of yoga and criticize it thoughtlessly.

The serious student of holistic yoga must bear in mind that yoga is a way of life. It is not a cheap miraculous pill that you can get from a guru that will solve all your problems. First of all, one must have a desire to live in a healthy body and to enjoy all the good things of life. It takes a personal discipline to achieve this goal. Usually people come to yoga for many reasons, and the holistic yoga offers something for everyone. If you are suffering from depression, anxiety, or serious psychological problems, you should first seek the help of a mental health professional before starting the practice of holistic yoga. Although the first lessons of hatha yoga will be beneficial for anyone with any emotional conditions; for further advanced stages of yoga a guru or a well-trained yoga instructor is necessary. The goal of yoga is to achieve a balanced mind in a healthy body.

It has been stated in the beginning of this introduction that yoga is already in you. Then a person in distress who has read about yoga could ask why yoga is not helping in her life. The following example could answer this question: Suppose you are living in a cold room. It is so cold you feel that your blood is freezing and your whole body is shaking. But in the corner, there is a beautiful fireplace with plenty of wood and matches. You are so lazy that you do not have the energy to light it up and to make fire for your own good. Then whom do you have to blame? No one but yourself. To make yoga useful, you have to light it up in your own body and keep nurturing it regularly, so it does not burn out.

About laziness, I shall tell you a tale well-known in India. There was a man who was so lazy that he would not even make an effort to cook his own food. He would beg for food from house to house, whenever he could get it. One day he was travelling on foot in a village. On the way he was so hungry that he could not continue, so he stopped under a mango tree, which was full of ripe mangoes. He laid himself under the tree and mangoes started falling near him. He opened his eyes and was asking for help. A mango fell near his mouth; he just turned his head and opened his mouth to eat it. He could not even lift up his hand to take it.

The beauty of the science of yoga is that you can achieve what you want, but you have to make an effort. There is an old saying: help yourself and God will help you. In this world, there are people who say they believe in God; however, they remember the Lord only when they are in distress—when they are suffering from diseases, financial difficulties, or upheavals in their lives. As soon as their situations improve, with more financial security, they forget about God. If they are not lucky enough and their prayers remain unanswered, they lose faith in God.

Others say they don't believe in God, but as soon as they are affected by calamities, they call upon the Lord for divine intervention.

The yogi knows that he or she is a small fragment of God, and within that small fragment all the good qualities of the Lord are virtual. Therefore, she is a blessed creature who can be happy, fully enjoy life, while waiting for the final liberation to unite with the Lord.

Is it not written in the Bible that man was created according to the image of God? Did not Lord Jesus say that, "I and my father are one and you also will be on my right side to share with me His kingdom?" Then why should we think that we are all born sinners, and there is no way to purify ourselves, therefore we are doomed to suffer a negative karma?

Why is there so much hatred and violence in our society, and all over the world? Why some fanatic groups are using religion to terrorize others? Why the rich always want more and will not hesitate to take the last penny of the poor? Why some powerful leaders, when taking office, think first of their own interest, instead of the welfare of the people? Why stronger nations think that their way of life or their culture is superior to the weaker nations? The selfish behavior is not necessarily innate; it develops through the process of nature and nurture. That is a personal characteristic. Integrity and spiritual aspiration develop according to several factors, including psychological, emotional, and one's view of societal rules and justice.

Every morning, the sun rises up and spreads its rays equally upon everybody, whether good or bad. The problem remains in man who does not know himself, who is not self-controlled, and who is a permanent trouble-maker for himself and for others. Every one of us is aware that life is short and there is no guarantee how many years one will live and when one will depart from this earth. However, many people behave like they are immortal, and they own the world. We are living in a tech society in this 21st century, where brilliant minds have created marvelous products to make our lives more comfortable. However, the vast majority of living beings have little knowledge of themselves. The science of yoga which starts with the body will help us to understand our place in the universe.

The philosophy of yoga is theistic, though it is not a religion. A religious-minded person is not necessarily a believer in God. As we know, throughout history and even currently many atrocities are committed in the name of God. Religion is a man-made idea to bring a group of people under control, while faith in a Supreme Being is an inner feeling which brings happiness, peace, divine love, and hope in a better life to come.

A yogi or yogini has the right and the full choice to believe in any form of God his or her imagination can think of. In the Hindu mythology, there are thirty-three million forms of God, though they believe in one Supreme Brahma (God). In India, you can see in one temple some devotees are worshipping their ideas of God in the image of Shiva. In another one, somebody else is worshipping Kali Mata, or in a third temple a lady is worshipping the image of Krishna. However, no one will feel that his or her idea of God is superior to the other worshiper or try to convert one another or to start a fight. On the contrary, as soon as a devotee of Shiva has finished worshipping her Lord, if on her way home she comes across a temple of Krishna or other images of God, she will also bow down and pay her respect to them. This is the old transcendental thought that God is everywhere, omnipotent and omnipresent.

Everyone has the right to live in peace. So, our duty is to struggle for peace through our own example of tolerance and universal love. In doing so, we can inspire our children and new generations to become better members of society. Daily yoga practice leads to self-control and peace within. When one has achieved peace, there is no need to disturb the neighbors. If all the nations' rulers and leaders were self-controlled yogis and yoginis, don't you think that the world would have been a better place? The common people are just like foot soldiers in an army, who are following the orders of their superiors. It is up to the rulers by their own living example of wise leadership to make a better world for all. I must acknowledge the wisdom of the current leader of India (Prime Minister Narendra Modi, a practitioner of yoga), who has made yoga at the core of the development of India. We have seen frequently and at certain occasions in New Delhi and other cities, government employees, soldiers, university students, and the public involved in mass yoga exercise and meditation by the thousands. Such mass yoga gathering also happens all over the world during International Yoga Day. On December 11, 2014, the United Nations General Assembly (UNGA) adopted a resolution which was approved by 177 countries, declaring June 21 International Yoga Day (Ban Ki-moon, UN Secretary General, 2015).

In the Puranas (yogic scriptures) is written the following basic teachings of yoga: Ahimsa (non-injury), Satya (truthfulness), Asteya (absence of stealing), Brahmacharya (sexual control), Aparigraha (absence of greed), and Saucha (Purity), Santosha (contentment) etc.... as Niyama. According to those Puranas, the *sadhakas*, or adepts of yoga, unless these rules of morality are observed, full success in yoga is deemed impossible.

From this statement of the yogic scriptures, you can understand that besides the commonly known physical exercises of yoga, there is something deeper in it. If you are just exploring the science of yoga, do not feel frightened by the teaching of the Puranas. You should not say to yourself that you cannot observe all of those rules and therefore yoga is not for you.

In all developing or developed countries, children must start school at about the age of five. But all will not reach the level of the university or become post-graduate students. However, at least all should know their alphabet, be able to read and write in order to become better citizens and productive members of society. What is important for the new seeker of yoga is a desire to keep the body healthy and a sound mind, in order to enjoy life. To reach the supreme goal of yoga will depend on everyone's own spiritual talent and karma.

In the same way, it is not necessary for everyone to hold a Ph.D. diploma in order to make a living and to feed the family. So, it is also not necessary for you to become a fully realized yogi in order to be in good health and to enjoy a peaceful harmonious life with your loved ones. In a bottle of five gallons, can you put ten gallons of water in it? Only a foolish, mentally ill person will try to do that. Similarly, in yoga you should not try to go beyond your own capacity.

In the yoga tree, there are many branches of yoga. This book is dealing with the entire tree. In the following chapters, various forms of yoga philosophy will be discussed. The seeker of holistic yoga is also knowledgeable about the entire Indian literature of self-realization. The study of Vedanta philosophy, the *Bhagavad Gita*, the Upanishads, etc. are all elements that the yogis use to arrive at self-realization. In Vedanta, which can be classified under Jnana yoga (intellectual knowledge), the body is not given much importance. The emphasis is on the philosophical reasoning about God. The body is considered as an illusion, *maya*, though it is visible to the naked eyes. It is seen as a mass of impurity, which is the result of one's own karma. No discipline is prescribed for the body in the form of exercises in order to keep it in good shape. The philosophy of Vedanta is mostly intellectually-based—that is, the study of scriptures, hymns, ritual, and repetition of mantras. This practice is supposed to be sufficient to keep the mind in tune with God's vibrations.

The goal of this book is not to give you a secret theory of yoga which will make you a Superman or a Wonder Woman. It is to inform and to encourage all yoga enthusiasts that the wonderful body we are born with should not be considered as a burden, a source of misery and unhappiness. You have the opportunity and the possibility to develop the yoga within through a simple lifestyle change, in order to achieve good health and happiness you deserve.

Many books have already been written on the yoga subject by eminent scholars, gurus, or pundits. The goal of this book is not to add one more on the library's shelves, but it is to bring to the benefit of all my own testimony based on personal experiences about the ancient science of yoga, which is today so popular in Western countries.

During my first years of yoga practices in India, many of my guru's brothers and teachers asked me to write about my meditation experiences. I always refused by telling them that I have got nothing much to say about it. Twenty-five years ago, I started writing about yoga, but I kept the manuscript in a drawer. It is just recently, after more than forty-five years of regular yoga meditation, that I decided to write this book. I am a yogi, also a psychologist, and I have always been scientifically-minded. I never used to accept anything blindly but had to test it. It is for this reason, while I was living previously in India during my search for truth, some gurus whom I met and who were surrounded by many faithful disciples, have considered me as a disobedient, unfit seeker, because I touched their hidden ego by asking too many questions.

In India there are many gurus dressed in red robes who are usually after name and fame. In order to get accepted, one must surrender blindly to them, like everybody else, without asking any questions. You will be told that the guru will do the thinking for you, and all you have to do is to obey him or her word by word, and you will get the blessings which will solve all your problems. A man like me, who believes in freedom and who always feels that nobody can give me anything without a personal effort, could never accept the thought of such masters.

However, in the mysterious Himalayas, there are also some hidden masters who are very simple and who may dress themselves as anybody else. Usually they have no disciples or have one or two devotees around them. If you have good karma and are lucky enough, you might be directed to meet such yogis. They can guide a seeker without any condition, if they feel you are sincere, unselfish, and qualified for deep yoga knowledge.

I was born and was raised in a very orthodox Catholic family. Every day, morning, noon, and at night, before taking food and retiring to bed, we all had to recite our prayers and intone some verses of the Bible, which we were supposed to have memorized. If some of us were already in bed, my father would awaken us to fulfill the daily routine prayers. Though since my childhood I was spiritually minded, I always felt that there is a connection between the body, the mind, and the feelings for God. I used to unknowingly do yoga postures in the bed, standing on my head, lying on my back, and pushing my legs toward the head; and I was feeling good. I always was an open-minded person. I never felt guilty for going to a Protestant or an Adventist church or to some other Christian sect, though if my father knew about it, he would have punished me. I always felt that God is everywhere and mostly wherever people of good will are praying.

Haiti is my native place and Voodoo is a common religion, mostly among the masses. I also used to attend with some friends to some Voodoo ceremonies whenever I got a chance. After attending, I went to my church at the confessional room; I never confessed that to the priest, because I did not feel guilty.

The science of yoga is indeed a practical technique, and the yogic scriptures are considered just like a huge map which gives only information about the area. Suppose you have not seen California before and you wish to go there. You can take a map and from it you may gather a lot of information about California. However, the map will not tell you of what kind of show is advertised for tonight at the street's corner theater, or if there is a policeman directing traffic. If you want to know all of that, you will have to go there and find out for yourself. It is the same for yoga. Mere talk, discussions, and reading will not satisfy a true seeker. Only the practice of it can convince you of its effectiveness to achieve your goal. That is what I have been doing. I am practicing yoga meditation naturally for almost fifty years, and I love it. I have become addicted to it and it is necessary to my body in the same way as food, and my mind is well-balanced.

In the following chapters, a great portion of the book will be reserved for a practical study of hatha yoga in twelve lessons, in all of its different aspects. The goal of the <u>first part</u> of the lessons is to give you some practical advice, to remind you of some preliminary notions about anatomy and physiology, and to teach them through the light of yoga, for a better understanding of how the chakras in the body work. As we know, the human body is complex, and each yoga posture has a particular effect on the internal organ targeted.

The <u>second and third parts</u> of the book will explore many different yoga approaches. At the end, Raja Yoga will be studied with a complete synthesis of all the yoga approaches, which will be called *Psychology of Daily Holistic Yoga and Self-Realization.*

At the end you will learn that there are two kinds of yoga, one is <u>exoteric</u> and the other is <u>esoteric</u>. The exoteric yoga is the one which can be written on paper and explained in theory. For the esoteric yoga, I can only give you an idea and point it out to you in the far distance. It will be up to you, in order to increase your limited vision, to take a telescope and try to find out what it is all about.

Lauture Massac, Ph.D. (Yogi Darshan)
2016

TABLE OF CONTENTS

Lesson 3 Part 2
The Science of Pranayama
Rhythmical Pranayama with Retention (Kumbaka)
Retention with Empty Lungs
Lesson 43 Part 3
Higher-Yoga: The Way to the Discovery.
Concentration (First Step toward Meditation)
Concentration on one object
Visualization
Mental concentration on one idea
Mind emptiness

Lesson 4 Part 1
The moral code in yoga (Yama Niyama)
Lesson 4 Part 2
The Asanas (Postures)
12 Advices to the Sadhaka
The angle posture (Konasana)
Swastikasana (Swastika posture)
Halasana (Plough posture)
Vistrita Pada Sarvangasana (Spread out feet and limbs posture)
Gomukhasana (Cow head posture)
Setvasana (Bridge posture)
The great prayer posture (Bhunamanavajrasana)
Dhanushasana (Bow posture)
The alternative of breathing or (Anulum Vilum)
Lesson 4 Part 3
Higher-Yoga: Meditation
The practical technique of meditation
The contemplation

Lesson 5 Part 1
Preliminary notions on muscles and articulations
Superior muscles of the limbs
The articulations
Lesson 5 Part 2
The postures (asanas)
The triangular postures (Konasana and variants)
The bent tree posture (Vakrikrita Vrikshasana)
Other variants of Matsyendrasana
The cow posture (Bhadrasana)
Pranayama: The alternate breathing with retention
The cool waves pranayama (Shitali)

The Cosmic Breathing

Lesson 11 Part 1
The action of Yoga upon the spinal column
Lesson 11 Part 2
The Asanas
The half leg posture (Ardha Padasana)
On the toes postures
The lotus posture
The lion posture in lotus (Padmasinhasana)
Great prayer posture in lotus (Bhunamana Padmasana)
Fish posture (Matsyasana)
The science of breathing nostril (Pranayama)
Ear Pranayama
Lesson 11 Part 3
Higher-Yoga: The Yoga of the New Age (Karma Yoga or Selfless Loving Services)

Lesson 12 Part 1
The action of Yoga upon the entire human complex system
Effects upon the articulations and the muscular system
Effects upon the digestive system
Effects upon the circulatory and respiratory system
Effects upon the nervous and endocrine system
Lesson 12 Part 2
The Asanas
The complete wheel posture (Purnachakrasana)
The shaking posture (Lolasana)
Variant of the coq posture (Kkutasana)
The mountain posture (Parvatasana)
Vertical lotus posture (Urdhvapadmasana)
Lotus in Halasana posture (Shirshasprushta-Padmasana)
Abdominal retraction in lotus (Uddiyana Bandha-Padmasana)
Half tied lotus posture (Ardha Baddha Padmasana)
Complete tied lotus posture (Baddha Padmasana)
The science of breathing (Pranayama); the feeding Pranayama
Double retention pranayama
Lesson 12 Part 3
Higher-Yoga: The Way to Immortality.

.

CHAPTER I

THE CONCEPT OF THE GURU

Since yoga has been in existence in India, it has been a great necessity to seek first a *guru* (spiritual master) in order to learn the science of yoga. In ancient time, the masters used to live in isolated places near the banks of rivers, in forests, or in the mountains with their disciples. Those masters were real, enlightened beings with deep knowledge of the yogic science. Many masters who specialized in different branches of yoga could be found in those isolated places.

During those days, the study of spiritual sciences was paired with the development of intellectual sciences. Everywhere—in cities, suburban areas, or in forests—many ashrams with their *gurukula* were to be found. *Gurukula* means *the place of the teacher* (Prabhupada Swami, 1970). In those gurukula, or schools for youngsters directed by the guru, besides the Sanskrit studies considered as a celestial language, the anatomical knowledge of the physical body was taught to the youngster through hatha yoga.

According to the guru, real knowledge is not possible without the control of the senses. One must know quite well the functioning of every organ, the limbs, and finally the mastery of the mind.

During those days, real success in life was not to gain great intellectual knowledge and to secure material wealth. A self-controlled and a balanced mind was the ambition of all seekers in order to live a harmonious life within themselves and nature.

The guru was the teacher who could show the way to achieve this goal. The aspirant could not think of starting with any spiritual discipline without the help of a guru. During those days, it was not difficult to find a guru, because it was the norm. Those great teachers were the guides of society and therefore were available to anyone who felt the need to have one for self-development.

Today in our modern civilization, to find a real and available master to teach the spiritual science is very difficult. It is even more difficult to find a true seeker who is fit to learn the knowledge from the guru. So instead of wasting precious time to search for a physical guru, one should start the search within. Various means are available to stimulate your inspiration: good yoga books, conferences, yoga centers, online spiritual yoga sites, etc. If you are not ready to meet the guru, you may have him just before your eyes and you will not be able to recognize him. Your unpurified mind will see in him or her an untrusted imposter, which could be the reflex of your own projection. Today in the 21st century, the masters do still exist physically or on a higher spiritual level.

We are living in a chaotic world with unceasing upheaval, which affects humanity—regional wars, terrorist attacks, refugee crises, school shootings, racial disturbances, and natural disasters. All of this could make the superficial observer think that the planet and humanity are dominated by negative forces, and therefore they are moving without guide and goal in the boundless cosmic space.

We can say that it is a mistake to believe so. On higher levels, the enlightened masters are permanently watching and directing the process of evolution, according to the divine projects, invisible except for those advanced souls who can sometimes in meditation penetrate into their divine surroundings. Some of their younger brothers are sent physically from time to time to different parts of the world to guide and inspire the sincere seekers.

Those great beings who have gone through the human process in many births have reached perfection. However, due to love, they have renounced the blissful state of nirvana in order to guide suffering humanity, while remaining invisible. Without their guidance, humanity would have proceeded towards its goal blindly.

The guru works for the welfare of mankind on two different levels. As an older brother or sister, he or she assumes a physical form, remains among seekers, and helps them on their journey to spiritual realization. In a transcendental way, the guru remains invisible in order to guide advanced adepts on the spiritual path.

WHAT IS THE DIFFERENCE BETWEEN A PHYSICAL GURU AND AN ORDINARY PERSON?

A physical guru is apparently an ordinary person, who by the grace of God and his positive karma has worked his way out of human darkness. From previous births, he already has purified a great portion of his physical and mental body. In this present birth, he is at the end of his purification work, and therefore is quite different from the ordinary person. Physically there are not many differences between him and the common man. In the same way you cannot tell the difference between a scientist and a simple illiterate laborer. Physically they both look like human beings, but intellectually there is a great difference. You can know the difference only when they start talking or exchanging ideas. For an advanced being, it is still more difficult to find out about his or her realization, because it is more spiritual (hidden) than intellectual. The difference can only be felt by sensitive, sincere spiritual people, and if some time is spent in the surroundings of such a master.

If it was so easy for all to recognize an advanced guru, the greatest divine master who came to earth in the physical body of Jesus would have been recognized by all, and the great tragedy we know would have been avoided. Even those who were supposed to be enlightened teachers during that time could not see in Him a divine being, although according to the Bible, His behavior in society was compassionate, rightful, and impartial. He demonstrated His miraculous powers to feed the hungry, to cure diseases, and even to raise the dead, and was still rejected. Of course, during those days, there were some great souls who could feel His divinity. But their views were not the views of the majority, and because of Him, they were persecuted and labeled as dangerous fanatics. That is why in the yogic scriptures the concept of *Yama-Niyama* (purity, selfless services to humanity) is prescribed for successful self-realization. This concept will be discussed in detail in subsequent chapter.

It is difficult for saintly persons to move around sinners unless they have a special mission. Otherwise, the advanced masters prefer to work in their invisible form for the welfare of humanity, to avoid any unnecessary persecutions which could compromise their spiritual work. Their younger brothers are dispatched to earth for a closer contact with their fellow beings. They then will teach the **exoteric** aspect of the divine science in order to prepare the heart and the mind of man for higher transcendental knowledge.

If you want to experiment with the notion of purity (cleanliness) and the notion of being filthy, dress yourself in clean white clothes and go and stay in a place where all are dressed in dirty clothes, with filthy behavior. When you arrive there, you will at once notice their unsanitary look, because you are cleanly dressed. Now try to approach them gently and open a civilized conversation with them. They will feel that you don't belong there. Instead of imitating you by washing themselves, they will try to soil your white garment by throwing all kinds of dirty things at you. From this simple experiment, you may have a better idea of the problems of an enlightened guru who wishes to help his brothers and sisters.

There is another experiment you can do with yourself to understand the difficult task of a living advanced teacher among human. Suppose you are having a very agitated life, with many wild friends who come to pick you up almost every night for all kind of enjoyments in night clubs. One day you tell your friends that you want to live a quiet life away from drinking, smoking, and you have found a spiritual discipline which has changed you. Invite them to join you and to share with you your new peaceful joy of life. You will see their reactions. They will call you a dreamer, a mad man, and think you have been brainwashed, and they will turn against you.

The true guru also, as long as he or she has a physical form, has to suffer and be humiliated because of his desire to teach equal divine love to all. His idea of showing the spiritual way which leads to peace and salvation is not always welcomed by all.

The seeker who wishes to develop spiritually must first understand the concept of the guru. Whatever you want to learn in life, you need a teacher. A real businessperson, in order to succeed in business, needs a teacher to teach him business administration. A doctor needs a teacher to teach him medical science. I am a classical piano player; I started to play at the age of seven, and I always had a teacher. Even today, I always feel the need to have a teacher to help me play better. In the spiritual field, one also needs a teacher, who is like a big brother to teach the salutary way to self-control and happiness.

It is stated in the yoga Upanishads that the guru is the way, he is the one who can give you whatever good things you need. The guru knows all the yoga paths very well. He or she will help you to tread the path safely, which is convenient to your own temperament. It is more difficult for an ordinary person to imagine or adopt a transcendental invisible guide as his guru. A physical guru who can inspire by his own rightful way of living could be the best support for any spiritual advancement.

The guru can be compared with a dynamo which will accelerate spiritual growth in you. Since every aspirant is different in his or her nature, the guru can customize a yoga path suitable to each individual. In many cases, it is very difficult to tread alone the **holistic** yoga path. The poor will of the aspirant is usually too weak to regularly maintain spiritual work. A novice yogi will very often get discouraged, due to his or her surroundings and various circumstances. If one does not have a guru, one sometimes can give up the practices and take different bumpy directions.

In this world, some people are born with a stronger will and more determination than others. Such people will succeed in whatever walk of life they have chosen. In society, they are the leaders, the responsible people, the directors of firms and institutions. In a way, they represent to others the gurus (guides). With their thoughtful guidance, their firms or institutions will function properly. All employees or subalterns have to follow the policy implemented by the director or the guide. If the guide is not regularly at his or her post, the subordinates are not receiving proper directions and many errors could jeopardize the whole operation of the company.

The only difference with a spiritual guide (guru) is his unbiased or impartial love toward all. He is a loving guide, not a commander. He is guiding the seeker without any personal gain. He does not expect anything in return from anybody, not even gratitude. If the seeker is naturally a grateful soul, it is good for him. Such quality will help her to progress on the spiritual way and to better serve humanity. However, the guru should have no concern with that. His duty is to serve and to help whenever he has the opportunity.

If a guru expects gratitude from a follower, he will often be disappointed because the disciples are still ordinary people, but of course with the difference of having a higher grade of inner search desire. Their willpower is feeble and can therefore make the mind unstable. A seeker whose mind is not regularly focusing on the practice of the teaching of a guru can, in a feeble moment of negative influence, give up the whole search for a lower idea. So, if a guru keeps nurturing the hope of gratitude from his disciples, he will be deceived many times. If the greatest divine guru, Lord Jesus, was expecting to taste the fruit of His work among His followers, He would have been much disappointed, and at the time of His death would not have said, "Father, forgive them; they don't know what they are doing."

A yogi aspirant who comes to yoga and wishes to conduct within the self a deep inner search is quite sincere in the beginning. However, the circumstances of his negative surroundings can influence his weak mind and compel him to make unwise changes in his or her views of life. Only a deep, sincere, divine love can save such a person from falling off the path. During that challenging period, the renewed spiritual energy of the guru is needed to pursue the journey.

DIFFERENT TYPES OF GURUS

To learn the yogic spiritual science, one can find many different levels of gurus. Some are specialized in the yoga philosophy of Vedanta, in hatha yoga, in bhakti yoga, or in purna yoga, etc. All of those specialized gurus are great and valuable masters. However, there are still differences in the quality of the teaching they can impart into a *sadhaka* (student).

A pandit guru, or a learned man, will be able to teach the Vedanta philosophy to a seeker. In the Vedanta philosophy, the body is given less importance; whether diseased or healthy, the intellect is the main vehicle, which needs to be transcended to arrive at divine knowledge. The body is considered as illusory (*maya*); it is like the clothes one is wearing every day—when it is dirty or worn out, it needs to be changed. In this path, the aspirant must climb to the spiritual heights with the help of his mind and intellect. Through philosophical reasoning one is supposed to solve the mind\body problems, and consequently lead the mind to a state of transcendental meditation. (Bevalkar, S.K. 2006).

A Hatha Yogi guru will teach all aspects of physical yoga. This is the opposite of Vedanta philosophy. According to hatha yoga, the body is the best instrument which will lead the seeker through self-realization, so the aspirant must be fully aware of the anatomy and the right functioning of his internal organs.

A Bhakti Yogi guru is a very emotional being. He has surrendered his will to the Supreme Lord, so he or she will not prescribe any special technique to a sadhaka. His path is devotional, and he remains in harmony within himself and the cosmic energy by singing spiritual songs and repeating prayers or mantras.

The Karma Yogi guru will teach salvation through social work. In this yoga concept, and according to the guru, personal salvation is not real. The whole of humanity must reach the divine blissful state at the same time. Without unselfish service to society, no religious practices, no yoga or meditation can lead one to self-realization. According to the guru's teachings, karma yoga is the best way to prepare the mind, body, and spirit for higher knowledge.

DIFFERENT TYPES OF ASPIRANTS

Many aspirants wish to have a first-class enlightened guru, but they do not ask if they, themselves, are truly first class sadhakas.

An ordinary aspirant is someone who is usually unstable in his or her ideas. She will start learning one subject, and after a short period of time she will give it up for something else. Such an aspirant is often very critically minded. She will go from ashram to ashram, guru to guru, and will criticize the ashrams and find defects in all the gurus. Even in ordinary loving relationship, he or she will go from boyfriend to girlfriend; and each deception will create a momentary sorrow in the heart, which will make her seek further spiritual guidance.

After seeing so many gurus, reading so many books, and going to so many different spiritual places or yoga centers, the sadhaka at the end will either follow a charlatan guru or give up the practice. Such category of aspirants enjoys the company of the guru who will teach the easy way, the one who preaches that one can be happy and obtain salvation in this birth without any unhealthy or destructive lifestyle changes.

The guru who tells his followers, "You can meditate and realize yourself, it is not necessary to give up your actual lifestyle. Keep eating as much red meat as you want. It is not necessary to give up smoking or drinking. Enjoy your body as you please, you will get liberation anyway."
—such gurus are very successful among ordinary aspirants, because most people do not want any drastic changes which will disturb their lifestyle,

even if it is beneficial to them. Perhaps you remember seeing a commercial on weight loss on TV directed toward obese people who are trying to lose weight, but who love to eat. They claimed with their diet method, you can eat as much pizza as you want, ice cream, and anything you desire. You are guaranteed to lose weight. Well, many obese people believe that and order their product, because it is the easy way.

If a magic pill which promises peace, happiness, and self-realization could be found in the stores, such stores would be constantly running out of supply. So, an ordinary aspirant will get the guru he or she deserves. (At the end of the book, all those different yoga methods will be studied and discussed in the chapter reserved for the synthesis of the holistic yoga.)

A medium type of aspirant is the one who feels the need for a deep spiritual search in his heart. He or she is religious-minded. He likes to go to church of his own religion. He is dogmatic-minded and likes to take the remarks of his bishop or pastor and the writings of holy scriptures. When he comes to yoga, because of his religious dogmatic ideas, he may have the feeling of changing religion, though he will find in yoga similar principles of divine love taught by the worshiped guide of his religion, (such as Jesus, Buddha, or Mohammed, etc.). He likes to combine worldly enjoyments and spiritual practices. He does not feel comfortable with a guru who suggests any kind of hard discipline. Gold must be in his right hand and God's knowledge in his left hand. He may follow for some time the teachings of a guru, and after a few months or perhaps a couple of years, switches over to another one. He will, however, maintain a steady spiritual search. He is comparable to the ordinary aspirant.

If he is able to develop the impartial spiritual love in his heart, he will surely come to understand the subtle aspect of spirituality, and probably will become a fit yoga sadhaka. He or she will get the deserved guru who will help prepare the way. After experimenting with various religions, gurus, and spiritual disciplines, he will finally find a new guru, or go back to the previous one. Such aspirant will be among the most faithful and sincere seekers.

The superior aspirant is a gifted sadhaka with many natural high qualities. He or she is generous, open-minded, truthful, young in heart, sincere, and has a balanced mind, with a mystical nature. He comes to the guru not to test his knowledge or to criticize him or her, but to follow his living example. He is unattached to material things. He is always joyful and understands the problems or suffering of others. He likes to help, to serve, and to protect the weak whenever he has an opportunity to do so.

If he occupies a position in society, his integrity is solid. He does not like to show off, and his ego is under control. He will keep secret his spiritual practices and remain faithful to his guru. He will be among the successors who will continue the guru's teachings unselfishly to others. Such great soul is fit to have the best guru. When he is in the presence of a highly developed master, he will feel his vibrations. Because of his good karma or natural qualities, he will be able to see and feel the differences between the master and an ordinary person. He won't have to search any further for the master. He will just go directly to him. They will be attracted to each other. It is just like sugar which attracts the bees. The disciple is ready to learn, and the guru is ready to teach. The aspirant will feel that the guru is not a stranger to him or a boss, but a dear family member, a father or a mother who wants to help his beloved son or daughter.

In Western countries or in India, many gurus are available. You cannot say they are impostors or smart business people. Ask to yourself rather if it is right to go to them, and if you are fit to understand what they are teaching. Why a true guru should come out and start displaying to all his knowledge, if there is nobody fit to understand?

The concept of the guru is not found only in yoga. It is also in all religions and social bodies. A leader who is directing the subordinates represents a guru. If the gurus are making business at the cost of the followers, it is because that is what the followers deserved.

If you are sincere, with the right discriminating power, how can you be misguided by an impostor? No matter what branch of yoga you wish to follow, the first necessary step is a sincere desire and a full understanding of what you really want to achieve. If these two primordial qualities are in you, then it will be very difficult for you to accept copper for gold or the mask for the face.

A real guru will not make propaganda around him in order to attract disciples. On the contrary, you may find it very difficult to get close to him. If he has a mission which draws many people towards him and appears busy with all, you should not think that he is indifferent to you who wish to be his close, sincere disciple. You will have to work upon your ego and keep trying to meet him, no matter how many times his close associates will tell you that he is not available. When you will meet him, you will understand that he also wanted to meet you. Patience with an open mind is very necessary for a seeker to meet his guru. The behavior of a realized guru is so unpredictable that it is a mistake to judge him in advance.

Listen to the story of the great yogi Naropa (an 11 century Indian yogi), who wanted to meet his guru, Tilopa. Naropa was a Brahmin pundit who was strict with the rules of his caste. Though he was a learned man, well established in the Vedas and yoga Shastras, he always felt the need for a guru to show him the way to self-realization. One day he heard about the great realized guru Tilopa, so he decided to go and search for him. He arrived in a village where they said Tilopa was and asked for his whereabouts. Someone said that Tilopa was sitting near the bank of a river catching fish.

He began to doubt in his mind, and thought, *Is it the business of a guru to catch fish?* But his sincerity leads him to the bank of the river.

When he arrived there, he saw a man sitting near a fire roasting freshly-caught fishes and was then eating them. In his mind, he began to think that this man cannot be my guru, because he is eating fish, and I am a Brahmin. However, while thinking that way, he was astonished to see that every time Tilopa finished eating a fish, he threw the skeleton in the river and suddenly it became a live fish again.

When Naropa approached him and was ready to talk to him, the man vanished. Naropa was not ready to give up his search, so he kept asking everywhere for Tilopa.

In another village somebody told him that Tilopa was sitting at the stairway of a temple. He went there but found a dirty beggar. He starts thinking, *how could this dirty beggar be my guru? I am an upper-class Brahmin.* Then he went to him and asked him, "Are you Tilopa?"

The man laughed and vanished before his eyes.

Now Naropa began to say to himself, *I must find my guru, I do not want to die without the grace of an enlightened guru.* So he continued with his search. He arrived in another village and asked again for Tilopa. He was told that Tilopa was around there, but he went to meditate in a graveyard nearby.

He said "Oh! How could a guru meditate in a place as impure as a graveyard?"

When he arrived to the graveyard, he found a man sitting crossed-legged on a tomb. He asked him, "Are you Tilopa?"

The man laughed and vanished.

Now Naropa had decided to purify his thoughts and prejudices. He began to prostrate before anything which came on his way. He saw a dog and said, "This is Tilopa," Then he saw an old man and said, "This is Tilopa." Then a big banyan tree, and he prostrated under it and said, "This is Tilopa." At the end, since his mind was cleansed of all kind of prejudices, he found a poor beggar majestically sitting on a stairway of a temple. Naropa fell at his feet and said, "You are Tilopa, my guru."

The man said, "Yes, I am Tilopa," and took his sandal and slapped him in the face. At once Naropa was illuminated. That was a *shaktipata* initiation, which made Naropa became the great realized yogi he was.

From that story, we can understand that if a seeker is sincere, he or she will surely meet his guru. His sincerity will help him to get rid of his prejudiced thoughts which created in him a barrier to self-realization.

As it has been stated in the beginning of this chapter, the guru is a vital necessity for the aspirant in search of higher yoga. However, instead of searching for one, start purifying your heart and mind to develop true sincerity.

When you are ready, inevitably you will meet the guru you deserve. Naropa was a learned man, well-versed in the Vedas and the yogic scriptures; therefore, he was ready to conduct a deep search within. He had only to get rid of his dogmatic ideas of his Brahmin caste. Since he had a sincere desire for self-Divine knowledge and salvation, his sincerity strengthened his faith and determination.

In later chapters, you will find all the means, in the form of yoga lessons, which will help you prepare the body and the mind for an eventual meeting with your guru, if so desired. Do not delay in exploring the science of yoga within yourself. You will not regret this personal experience in your life.

CHAPTER II

THE PERSONAL SPIRITUAL SEARCH IN INDIA

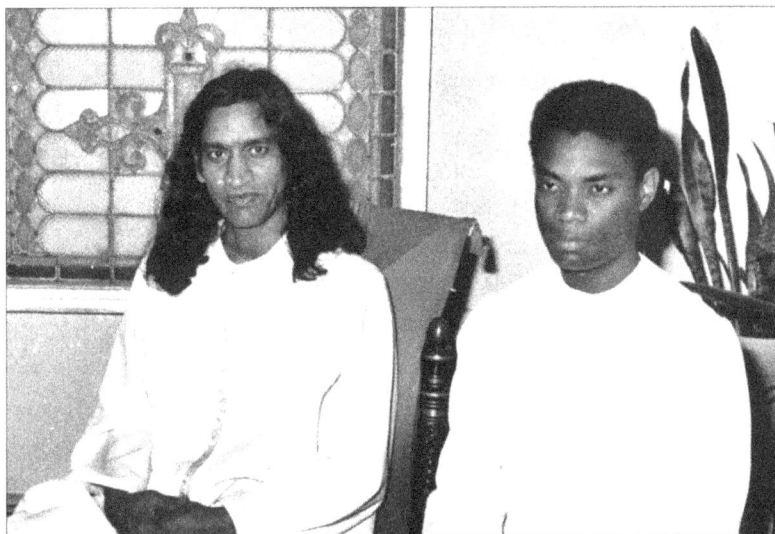

Yogi Amrit Desai and Dr. Lauture Massac (Yogi Darshan) at Kripalu Ashram, Pennsylvania, 1979.

The spiritual quest started when I was a teenager. I always felt a connection between the body and the mind. I was an avid reader of spiritual and scientific books. Within myself there always has been a desire for self-knowledge. I asked myself: *Who am I? Where did I come from?* and *What is the purpose of life? Is it to eat, to sleep, to procreate, and to die?* I wanted answers, and I was continuously searching for answers, just like an astrophysicist who is always searching the universe for new discoveries. I was blessed, because my quest for self-knowledge was a natural instinct. I always have a balanced mind, never feel lonely, depressed, or anxious. I was sociable, had friends, and liked to travel. Before I started my esoteric practice of yoga, I had a few relationships with women, but they never worked out; she always dumped me or I dumped her. I am a classical piano player. I had to practice several hours a day. And I am always busy. I never had any desire to smoke, to drink, or to use drugs. On the contrary, I felt that the body needs to stay healthy, and probably is the laboratory for my search. At the same time, this kind of spiritual quest was not religion-oriented. I never felt the need to be a priest, a monk, or a pastor.

At the age of 20, I started practicing yoga through the help of books I was reading. I also discovered the Theosophical Society and was fascinated in reading books of Mrs. Helena Blavatsky and Annie Besant, some founding members of the Theosophical Society (Gomes, M. 1987). After reading so many books about yoga, and practicing alone hatha yoga, I cherished the dream to one day go to the source of yoga in India to meet the masters I read so much about. Eventually in 1969, I went to India, and the first place I stayed was at the headquarters of the Theosophical Society at Adyar, Madras (presently known as Chennai) in South India. There, I met very interesting spiritual people. Every evening we had intellectual *satsang* (discussion about occultism and religions). The philosophy of the Theosophical Society welcomes everyone, whether you belong to a religion or you are agnostic. They have no dogma, no creed, are tolerant of others' beliefs, and are very friendly and loving; therefore, I was very comfortable in the company of such people.

From there, I shared my spiritual search plan in India with some people of the group, and I was given names of places of interest and spiritual masters. I added those names on a list of yoga masters I had to visit. Among them were: Maharishi Mahesh Yogi, Swami Muktananda, Dihlindra Brahmacharya, Satya Sai Baba, and others. There is another ashram I had on my list, which is the Shri Aurobindo Ashram directed by the successor of Shri Aurobindo, a French lady called "The Mother." The ashram is internationally known and is located in a town called Pondicherry, some 160 kilometers from Madras. Aurobindo was a yoga master whose teachings were based on the holistic yoga. He believed by surrendering to the Divine, one can discover the self. The Mother came from France to Pondicherry in 1914 to meet Aurobindo. They became connected to each other, and according to their writings and their followers, lived a divine life in the same house until Aurobindo's passing away in 1950. The Mother continued to live in the same house until her passing away in 1973. When I was in India in 1969, the Mother was still alive. I wanted to see her, and to try to understand the teaching, which consists of surrendering to the Divine Mother. Student residents at her ashram are not asked to practice any discipline. Each person must surrender to the Divine Mother and find his own way to achieve self-realization. No guidance is prescribed.

I spent four days at the Theosophical Society, and I was very pleased of my stay there. My discussions with open-minded spiritual people strengthened my determinations in my search for higher knowledge.

One early morning I took a bus to Pondicherry. Arriving at the ashram of Shri Aurobindo, I found a different atmosphere. It was like a small town, with everyone dressed like every ordinary Indian on the street. I did not see anyone dressed in red, like the monks I'd previously seen in ashrams. The place was like a commune; the residents worked at the ashram and lived nearby. In the afternoon, the Mother would show up to the balcony and give blessings to hundreds of devotees. That was the routine at this ashram. I spent two nights there and took a train to New Delhi.

Arriving in New Delhi, I took the bus to Rishikesh (one of the holiest places to Hindus, about 160 kilometers from Delhi). The bus made a stop for about an hour at Haridwar, another famous pilgrimage place, situated at the bank of the sacred Ganges River (or Ganga), the gateway to Rishikesh. When you arrive at Haridwar, you start feeling the spiritual vibrations of Rishikesh, which is only 20 kilometers away. I stepped out of the bus, washed my face, and collected holy water from the Ganga, which is few feet away from the bus stop. Soon we got back on the bus toward Rishikesh. Arriving at Rishikesh, you start feeling a cooler breeze compared to the heat at Haridwar, because it is situated at the foothills of the Himalayas, surrounded by the holy river of the Ganges. It is also known as the Yoga Capital of the World. Foreigners from all over the world come to this place to learn hatha yoga and meditation. In Rishikesh, you will find many temples and yoga ashrams. The most famous ashram is the Sivananda Ashram, the headquarters of the Divine Life Society, founded by Swami Sivananda, where he lived and died (in 1963).

Rishikesh is a pilgrimage place, and mostly during summer the place is crowded with tens of thousands of people. As soon as one arrives in Rishikesh, you can smell incense all over, hear the ringing bells of the temples, the sermons of the priests, and the chanting of the devotees over the loudspeakers. You can see monks dressed in red robes as well as beggars going up and down the streets. Naked sadhus, revered as saints, covered with ashes, with long, dreaded hair coiling on top of their heads, wander, and devotees pay respect at their feet. Sacred cows with painted red horns are roaming the street without being disturbed by anyone. The monkeys, some with babies under their stomachs, are jumping all over, looking to grab some food. They are considered as part of the human interactions. You can see constant movements of boats crossing the river, taking people from ashrams and temples on one side of the river to ashrams and temples on the other side.

The ashram of Maharishi Mahesh Yogi was on the other side of the river, so I took the crowded boat to go to see him. He was the guru of the Beatles (the famous British band) who came to see him in 1968, a year before I met him. I found the Maharishi seated, with a rose in his right hand and surrounded by many disciples, mostly foreigners. I approached him with respect. I listened to his discourse for several hours and left. I did not feel impressed or connected to him.

I spent two weeks at the Yoga Neketan Ashram, next door to Sivananda Ashram. There the accommodation was better, and foreigners could stay longer. While at the Sivananda Ashram, we could only stay a few days. During the day I attended yoga classes at Yoga Neketan, and silent meditation sessions in the evening with the guru swami. I also was going to Sivananda ashram three times a week in the evening for Satsang. The ashram always had a variety of events with invited guest musicians and dancers. One evening, I had the opportunity to listen to young Ravi Shankar (a famous Indian classical musician) playing the sitar. I also enjoyed the Vedanta lectures, mostly with the guru Swami Krisnananda (with whom I had several private meetings) and the Indian songs of bhakti yoga.

It is at the Sivananda Ashram where I met **Yogi Amrit Desai**. He came from America with a group of students. He was telling me about his guru, Swami Kripalvanandji, and invited me to come to Malav in the state of Gujarat, where he would be going next. I added the name of Kripalu to my list and wrote the direction of how to get to the ashram.

When I left Rishikesh, I went to visit Yogi Dhirendra Brahmachari in New Delhi with an Indian friend I met at Yoga Niketan, who had studied hatha yoga with him. He was telling me that his teacher was a great hatha yoga master, and I could learn many things from him. By the way, Dhirendra Brahmachari was the yoga teacher of Prime Minister Indira Gandhi. So, we took the train to New Delhi. We stayed in an ashram there, and the next day we were able to meet with Yogi Dhirendra at his residence. Physically, he was very impressive, with long hair, bearded, and piercing eyes with flat affect, looking like Rasputin (a Russian mystical faith healer). He was tall, slim, and dressed in a white robe with a *bindi* (red dot) on his forehead. When we arrived, he was sitting cross-legged on the floor in a large room with many foreigners, demonstrating hatha yoga and pranayama. He was performing very advanced yoga postures with some rapid breathing (Sahit Kumback). I participated in the session, and at the end I was introduced to him by my Indian friend and asked him several questions about the spiritual yoga. I didn't feel any connection, and I left a couple of hours later.

My next trip would be to Mumbai area, where I had on my list two places to visit. The first was Swami Muktananda in Pune, and next was the Lonavala Institute of Yoga. I heard about this yoga institute, where scientifically they were testing the claimed benefits of yoga, and they taught students about anatomy of yoga. So, I was interested to find out about this place and to learn something. From Delhi, I took the train to Mumbai, then a bus to Swami Muktananda's ashram located in a suburb of Pune. I did not have much money, but during those days travelling in India was cheap. I just got a third-class train ticket, and usually I stayed in an ashram, where everyone was welcomed for a short time with free food.

I arrived late in the evening at the ashram. I was welcomed with a glass of water (the usual Indian greeting) by one of his disciples and was assigned to a dorm with about 25 people, where I spent the night. The next morning at five o'clock, I heard bells ringing and people directing toward the temple where a puja ceremony was taking place. After the puja, the disciples went to do their Karma Yoga activities at their assigned position. Some went to the kitchen, others collected vegetables in the garden. I was hungry since I had not eaten anything for about 18 hours, but I did my yoga exercises and pranayama to get energy. I did not see yet Swami Muktananda. At around 11 a.m., I saw people going to the dining hall, and large leaves and metal cups were laid on the floor. We sat on the floor, and several cooks with baskets of bread (chapattis), buckets full of cooked vegetables and rice started serving us. Suddenly, I saw Swami Muktananda, half-dressed in a piece of red cloth, come in, take a basket of chapatti, and start throwing a chapatti at each person. I was impressed by his simplicity, because he was the first guru I saw in India who was serving people. The others were being served and appeared to enjoy being worshipped, as they pushed their hands forward to bless the devotees.

Swami Muktananda had a large ashram, and bus load of devotees were coming daily to the ashram, mostly from Mumbai. It appeared that he was not giving private audience. He was sitting in the meditation hall, which was crowded with about 300 people conducting kriya yoga. I spent three days at the ashram and I never had a one-on-one with him. I spoke many times to his close disciples who were telling me that Swamiji's teachings were mostly karma yoga to purify the seekers. When the seeker is ready, he will get *shaktipat* (the awakening). Although I thought that this guru was a kind and simple person, I did not seek to be a part of his teachings, so I moved on to my next spiritual adventure, which would be at Lonavala Yoga Institute.

I left the ashram early morning and took the bus to Lonavala, which is about 65 kilometers away. At around 11 a.m., I arrived at Lonavala. I met a yoga instructor who gave me a tour of the facility and explained to me what they do. He told me that people came there to relieve stress and hoped to cure some diseases through the scientific practice of yoga. He said they also had medical doctors who monitor the progress of the yoga practitioners. During my stay there, I learned how a hatha yoga posture affects a targeted organ of the body. I had the yoga teacher give me a demonstration on how he could slow down his heartbeat by doing a *pranayama* (breathing exercise). I learned the six kriyas for cleansing the body, which are described in the Hatha Yoga Upanishad. They are: Neti, Dhauti, Nauli, Shanka Prakshalana, Kapala Bhati Pranayama, and Trataka. I will give a brief description of each kriya technique. However, any attempt to practice those kriyas alone could be very dangerous to your health. They should be learned only under the guidance of a knowledgeable experienced instructor.

Neti is a nostril cleansing technique using a special vessel with a spout (like a teapot). Warm salty water is put in the pot, and the student is putting water in one nostril and it comes out in the other. A wet cloth string is also pushed in one nostril and comes out in the other. The benefit of this kriya is to cleanse the sinuses, relieve headaches, and strengthen vision.

Dhauti is cleansing of the esophagus and the stomach. A strip of cotton cloth approximately two inches wide and nine feet long is first dampened in warm salty water. Then it is slowly swallowed to the stomach. After a few yogic movements of the stomach, it is pulled out, usually with yellow phlegm. The benefits of it are to relieve acidity, to cleanse the esophagus and the stomach in order to increase digestive power.

Nauli is the churning or pumping of the stomach muscles. The benefit of it is the stimulation of the digestive system.

Shanka Prakshalana is the master of all the kriyas. It is the complete cleansing of the colon and the intestine. Usually the yogi practices this kriya once every six months. It is a natural, provoked purge to eliminate the toxins in the body. That is all I can say about its description.

Kapala Bhati Pranayama: With the head bending in right or left position, the student takes a deep inhalation through the mouth and exhales rhythmically with strong bursts through the nose several times. The benefits of this kriya are to cleanse the sinuses, to enhance breathing capacity, relieving stress, and to facilitate meditation.

Trataka: In this kriya, the student sits in meditative position in front of a candle. The eyes are kept open, gazing at the light without blinking for a couple of minutes. Then close the eyes and focus internally. This kriya is repeated several times, with increase of retention time. The benefits are strengthening of the eye muscles, and the development of mind concentration.

At the yoga institute, I learned safely the exoteric aspects of hatha yoga with experienced yoga masters. Now I was really feeling the need for transcendental knowledge. Despite the food condition I was getting (not eating on time the vegetarian diet), I felt that I was getting energy from someplace else. I thanked God for my young healthy body, and I felt that my body was the laboratory where I could discover what I was looking for. I had spent six days at Lonavala, and I was moving on to my next scheduled place.

MEETING WITH SWAMI KRIPALU AT MALAV ASHRAM

One early morning in the month of July 1970, from Lonavala in the state of Maharastra, I took the train to the state of Gujarat via Baroda. My destination was Malav ashram, situated in a remote small village some 50 kilometers from Baroda. It is where Swami Kripalu was living. From the city of Baroda, I took a bus to Malav. Even though the distance to Malav ashram was only about 50 kilometers, it took four hours to get there, due to the condition of the road at that time. Arriving at Malav in the afternoon, I was greeted by Swami Sutanand Muni, the manager of the ashram and the closest disciple of Bapuji Kripalu. Compared to other ashrams I had visited; this remote ashram was a small place. Besides the monk Swami Sutanand, dressed in red, no other monk lived there. Bapuji had many devotees from all over Gujarat who visited the ashram very often, but had no other disciples living with him. Bapuji Kripalu had his separate enclosed place, secured by a little gate. The swami told me that Bapuji was in meditation and came out in the mornings only for a short time to give *darshan* (blessings).

The next day, after doing all my yoga routine, I was asked to come out for breakfast. At about ten o'clock, the swami told me that Bapuji had come out. He took me to the gate, and as soon as I approached the gate I could feel the serenity of the place amid the divine smell of incense. Bapuji was seated alone on a swing, dressed in the regular red garment of the Indian swamis. I approached him and respectfully prostrated, and he raised his right hand, indicating a blessing sign. Swami Sutanand introduced me to him and told him that I came from America in search of yoga knowledge. Bapuji smiled, took a slate (since he was a silent monk) and wrote that I was welcome to stay. Whenever Bapuji came out, many people in the village also came for darshan. I sat in his company for a half hour and then we all were asked to leave.

The next morning, the same routine; Bapuji was again outside on his swing. I was the first one to get in there with the swami. This time I had many questions to ask. Swamiji was an educated man and was fluent in English. He translated my questions from English to Hindi. Most of my questions were related to yoga. As Bapuji was writing on the slate and the Swami was translating, I wanted to know more. Finally, Bapuji wrote "Beta (my son), If you want to stay here, you can stay." To that, I replied, "Yes, I would like to, but I am touring India and have a list of other masters to visit." Bapuji replied, "Go. If you are not satisfied, you can come back."

LEAVING MALAV ASHRAM - THE SEARCH CONTINUES

I spent five days at the Malav Ashram, and one morning I took the bus to Baroda and a train to Ahmedabad. I spent two nights with an Indian family in Ahmedabad, and then I proceeded to the city of Indore, in the state of Madhya Pradesh in search of yogis. My destination was a small village called Amli, where supposedly a powerful yogi was living, as I was told. First, I must say that throughout my travelling in India, I have witnessed people demonstrating some strange powers. Those people are called *fakirs* (wonder-worker), others are said to be practicing *Jadoo* (black magic). For example, in the West we see magicians performing on stage with all of their apparatuses. We know that they are earning a living by entertaining their audience with tricks. However, in India, when you see a fakir on the street, clothed in little more than loin cloths, with no sophisticated equipment, and he makes a mango seed grow three feet high with ripened mangoes, we don't know what to think. In a remote village, I was told that at about five o'clock in the morning, near the bank of the river in a special mystical ceremony, some people would be walking on fire. I said to wake me up early because I wanted to see it. The day before, they dug an 8' x 4' hole, about three feet deep, and filled it with trunks of wood. They let the wood burn for several hours.

After bathing in the river, I saw half a dozen garlanded men wearing loincloth, bare-footed and apparently in a trance-like state, walk slowly one by one on the red burning fire. I was approximately ten feet away from the fire, and the heat was intense. They were not doing it for money or for a show. I was told that it is a ceremony that takes place once a year at a specific date, to pay respect to a particular god.

Now to get back to my search for the yogi at Amli village. From where I got off the bus, I had to walk several hours. Usually I carried my own backpack, but this time it was too heavy on my back and I let my guide help me out. We finally arrived at the place where the yogi was staying. I saw a middle-aged man, disheveled, with long hair and wearing loincloth, seated cross-legged with two other sadhus in red garments in front of a small temple. The yogi spotted me, and I noticed that his eyes were fixated on me. I paid my respect to him, and he did not show any reaction. My guide did the talking, and the yogi was listening and did not say a word. We sat there for approximately 45 minutes. Suddenly the yogi stood up and left. This was the result of my long trip to this yogi. Later on, in my meditations, I will understand the importance of this silent encounter.

After this experience, I did not feel any desire to continue to visit other masters. I cancelled my trip to visit Satya Sai Baba's ashram. Now my mind was at Kripalu at Malav ashram. My guide went to the train station and arranged a ticket for me to Baroda. I took the night train, and the next day I arrived at Baroda. Again, from there, I took a bus to Malav Ashram.

Arriving at the ashram, I felt relief from this long trip. Swami Sutanand arranged to prepare food for me. At the ashram, there was a separate courtyard room across from Bapuji's enclosure. It is where I previously stayed, and I would be staying there again. Bapuji was in meditation, and probably I would be seeing him in the morning. The ashram was quiet; it was only the swami, kitchen devotees, and me.

Three days after my returning to the ashram, I suddenly experienced the awakening of kundalini power.

AWAKENING OF KUNDALINI POWER

I had been travelling all over in India for approximately three months. Now I felt that a sudden change was happening in my life. When I sat in meditation, automatic breathing was taking place, and I noticed that my body was automatically doing hatha yoga exercises. In other words, I was not able to do anything voluntarily; it was just like that I was possessed by a force that had taken over my body. I started singing and repeating mantras I had never heard.

Swamiji took me to Bapuji and explained to him what I told him was happening to me. Bapuji wrote on his slate to tell me to reduce my meditation time. Well, every time I sat and closed my eyes, that force was again taking over. Every day I was having different experiences. I was shouting, singing loud, and dancing. Bapuji could hear from his room my activities. In the ashram, they had not seen anyone manifesting this behavior in meditation. Swami Sutanand had been living with Bapuji for over six years and he had not experienced anything such as the awakening that I was experiencing. However, he was a very loving and knowledgeable man, and was very supportive of me.

As I was progressing, six days after the awakening my meditation was intense, with joyful transcendental experiences. I was not coming out of my room to eat, sometimes for ten hours. I was repeating *Ram Ram* mantras, uttering Sanskrit words that I did not know anything about. Since I was the first disciple at the Malav Ashram having those experiences, Bapuji was concerned for my psychological wellbeing and was asking me to stop the meditation. He thought that I was losing my mind. Mostly, because I was a foreigner, he did not want anything to happen to me under his watch. On my part, I understood exactly what was happening to me, and the whole meaning of the experiences I was having; therefore, I could not stop doing something which was so natural to me. Since I could not obey his order, I was asked to leave the ashram.

Sutari Muni, the manager of the ashram, who was a very kind, loving monk, said he would take me to a quiet place in another village about 75 kilometers away where I could do my sadhana. Indeed, the next day early morning, we took the bus toward a small village near the bank of the River Narmada called Sisodra.

PRACTICING MEDITATION IN SISODRA VILLAGE

We arrived at Sisodra in the afternoon. Swamiji introduced me to the village chief, who was one of Bapuji's devotees in the village. He let him know that I was Bapuji's *shisya* (student) who needed a quiet place to practice sadhana, and that they needed to look after me. The chief gathered a few devotees of Bapuji and they agreed to take turns in helping me with my daily needs. The chief said that there was an old abandoned bungalow on the hilltop near the bank of the river; he would get it for me. We went to see the bungalow. It was an old two-story house in the middle of a peanut field, with one room upstairs, an old concrete terrace, and three rooms downstairs, no bathroom. I was told that the house was a kind of shelter for wandering monks. In fact, one sadhu came to sleep in one room downstairs, and during the day he would go begging for his food.

I was delighted of this location. Since it was an isolated place, I imagined that I would be able to do my sadhana without disturbing anyone. I immediately chose the room upstairs. The devotees brought a couple of large clay containers for water on the terrace and other basic things for me. The house was walking distance to the river. I first went and bathed in the river, and returned back to the bungalow to enter into meditation. As soon as I sat down, the shakti went into action and I surrendered to it. The next morning at around six o'clock, I heard some movements on the terrace. I opened the door and I saw a big monkey opening the container and drinking the water. I chased him out, and I saw over a dozen monkeys, some with their babies under their bellies, eating peanuts in the field. It was early morning, and also all kinds of beautiful birds were flying and singing, looking for food. While observing the behavior of the monkeys and the activities of the birds, I felt more unity with all God's creatures in nature.

In my tenth day of the awakening of kundalini, I had no fear; I was living the presence of God in my own body. My entire search stopped. I had no need to search anymore for anything. I felt that within me there was an intelligent guide who was directing my actions and protecting me. I felt that ignorance had vanished, and the door of knowledge had been opened to me. I felt no need to read any books or to listen to any mortal being. An intelligent force was guiding and protecting me. Any action I did with my body, the meaning of the action was quite clear to me. When I was repeating a mantra or singing a song, I understood the reason for it. Later on, when I would get acquainted with the yoga Upanishads, I was amazed to read the descriptions of most of my experiences. Some are described in an esoteric way and could be understood only by an initiate.

After three months of safe practice of my sadhana, the Narmada River flooded the village. Many villagers evacuated with their livestock to the hilltop bungalow. All the rooms downstairs were full of people cooking, talking loudly, and taking care of their biological needs around the bungalow. I was surrounded with filth, fumes, and smell of tobacco. When the water receded, many people stayed because their huts where they were living washed away. They had no place to go. I decided to move out, and this time I headed toward Northern India.

PRACTICING MEDITATION IN THE HIMALAYAS

I was not on the move looking for gurus. I was, rather, looking for a quiet place away from people in order to develop my yoga knowledge. I took a train to Delhi, then a bus to Deladun. From Deladun, I took a bus to a holy place called Gangotri, which is high in the Himalayas. After several hours of dangerous ride through narrow curves in the mountain, I arrived in the village of Gangotri. The site is impressive, with a magnificent view of snow on the mountain. During the day the weather was pleasant, but it was somewhat chilly at night. Small temples are all over the place, and sadhus as well as devotees coming on pilgrimage perform rituals in the mighty river Ganges.

I located a cave near a temple. I organized myself and settled there to meditate. The vibrations of the place were very much conductive to my sadhana. I was a silent yogi, communicating with my helper on a slate. I was not eating much, living on chapattis (wheat flat bread) and cow milk offered to me by the villagers. Sometimes in a kind of samadhi, I spent hours bathing in transcendental lights with different indescribable color of light rays. In the cave alone, I had no fears, and I felt protected by the divine energy. Although one day walking in the jungle, I had a close encounter with a large cobra standing in front of me. I stopped and stared at it, and it flattened down and ran away.

I was progressing very well with my sadhana. One day I had the visit of a half-naked yogi. He entered the cave silently, and at once I recognized that I was visited by a divine being. He sat on the floor in front of me and projected his beautiful eyes to my eyes. I felt his energy, and it was like we were talking to each other. I entered into a trance. When I woke up, he was not there. Two days later, he came a second time and was radiating a golden light around his body. He stood up in front of the cave and lifted his hand and projected a ray of light to me. This time I was fully awake and bathing in the rays of light. He revealed to me some esoteric teachings and vanished. I never saw him again, but always felt in communication with him. I was living in the cave for the whole summer, but now winter was approaching, and it was getting very cold. I left the Himalayas and went to Mount Abu in central India.

MEDITATING IN MOUNT ABU

I arrived in Mount Abu in the month of December. There the weather was pleasant and cool at night. Through information I gathered from sadhus who had been to the area, I located a cave about a mile away from a temple. At first, I went to the temple where a pujari swami in charge was living. He told me that I could get my food from the temple. Every evening I had to go and collect my milk and chapattis (purchased) from the temple. The difficulty that I experienced is that every evening I had to walk a mile in the jungle to the temple. The swami told me that the milk was available after six o'clock, because there was a religious ceremony from 5 p.m. to 6 p.m. and the milk was offered to the god, and only afterward I could get it. I endured the situation for approximately three weeks. Walking in the jungle at night was very dangerous, but I had faith that I was protected. My meditation was going well in the cave, despite of my food problems.

Sometimes, I came out of meditation late, and was not able to walk that far and have time to come back before wild nocturnal animals came out in the jungle. Therefore, I told the religious swami that I was a yogi meditating in a cave and sending blessings to his temple. I told him that his god would not be offended if he could let me get the milk before the offering since I had to walk a long way in the dark. He immediately got mad and told me not to come back. I went to the village and purchased

34

my flour to make my own food. I lived there another three weeks on chapatti and water. Finally, I decided to go back to Bapuji Kripalu Ashram at Malav.

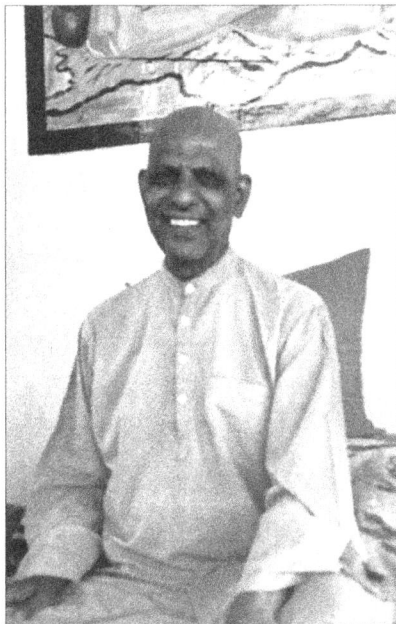

Swami Kripalvananda (Bapuji) at Kripalu Center, Pennsylvania, 1979.

RETURNING TO KRIPALU ASHRAM AT MALAV VILLAGE

When I arrived at Kripalu Ashram, Swami Sutananda welcomed me and assigned me the same bungalow where I had been meditating before. I briefly shared with him some of my ordeals throughout India in search of a suitable place to develop my sadhana. He told me to stay there and to stop moving around. In the meantime, he told me that Bapuji had been conducting shaktipat sessions for the first time since after my awakening at his ashram. In other words, I was the first sadhak who had been awakened into the kundalini knowledge at his ashram.

I met with Bapuji every day, and that was when he told me to learn Sanskrit and Hindi in order to understand first-hand the whole spectrum of the holistic yoga knowledge; and I did just that. Swami Kripalu was also known as Bapuji (respected father). Most Indian literature of sacred books are written in Sanskrit and translated into Hindi by eminent scholar yogis of ancient India. However later on, English translations from Hindi, mostly by Westerners, have not necessarily captured the esoteric essence of the original texts. That is why Bapuji was guiding me to go to the source in order to understand my experiences. However, before I started reading the yoga scriptures, everything was already crystal clear to me. The meaning of every *mudra* or yoga posture I was doing was clear to me. The books only confirmed and strengthened my faith in yoga.

I had a Sanskrit teacher who also was fluent in English and Hindi. I wanted to learn the yoga scriptures directly from the original, which are written in Sanskrit. So, I borrowed some yoga scriptures from Bapuji's library, and the teacher was translating the *slokas* to me. Within several months, I had consulted the following yoga scriptures with my Sanskrit teacher: Gheranda Samhita, Goraksa-Paddhati, Hatha Yoga Pradipika, Shiva Samhita, Patanjali Yoga Darshan, Siddha Siddhanta Paddhati, Yoga Yajnavalkya, and other yoga Upanishads. In listening to the translation of the sutras, I was delighted to see that yoga is a real science, because those books were written by yogis who have narrated their own experiences. Bapuji was a real yogi scholar, not a person with book knowledge. He meditated in silence ten hours a day, and during several years I spent near him I never heard him speak a word. When he came out of meditation, he answered my questions in writing on a slate. His personal library in the ashram was well-stocked with ancient yoga scriptures.

I mentioned earlier that Bapuji was conducting shaktipat initiation for the first time after my awakening at his ashram. That is where I met Swami Rajarshi Muni. At that time, he had not yet taken the vow of a swami. He stayed at the ashram, and a few days later took the red robe and became Swami Rajarshi. We were together at the ashram, and also Amrit Desai came back to the ashram, and both were interested to hear about my meditation and kundalini awakening experiences. Due to new meditation activities, too many people were coming to the ashram and I wanted to go away. That is when Swami Rajarshi Muni told me about a small village near Rajkot called Sapeur, where his parents lived in a quiet house. He said that he would make arrangements for me to stay with his parents to do my meditation. I gladly accepted and proceeded to Sapeur.

MEDITATING IN THE HOUSE AT
SWAMI RAJARSHI'S PARENTS AT SAPEUR VILLAGE

I arrived at Sapeur village in a small train, and Rajarshi's father was there at the station to meet me. He took me to his large old two-story home, located in a quiet place. I met his wife, and both introduced me to a room upstairs with a small terrace where I would be practicing my sadhana.

I organized myself and settled down in the place. Compared to Northern India, where it was cold during winter, in Gujarat and particularly in this area it was very hot, with no electricity or fan. Anyway, it was much better, since I had those wonderful people looking after me. Now I had been practicing kundalini yoga for approximately two years and I was progressing very well. As previously, I was keeping silence and communicating with Rajarshi's parents on a slate. They understood well and served me respectfully. I feel that I was in meditation all the time. However, I set a schedule for meditation in the morning from 8:00 a.m. to 12 noon, and in the evening from 4:00 p.m. until bedtime. Most of the time this schedule was not observed. Since I had surrendered to this yoga, sometimes I got absorbed in Samadhi all day and I didn't come out to eat. The wonderful state of yoga nidra (conscious dream state) I was in had transformed my circadian rhythms.

In this automatic esoteric meditation, every day I had different experiences. My daily routine was natural and at the same time transcendental. In whatever activity I was engaging (reading, playing harmonium and tabla), I was still in a meditative state. The days and months passed so fast, and one day I realized that I already had been meditating in this house for one year. From the revelations I received from the visiting yogi when I was meditating in the Himalayan cave, I understood that when the time came to go back to the West to spread the knowledge, I would receive a signal from him. In a meditation session I did receive his message, and I started planning to leave India to go to France. First, I went to Nepal for a couple of months, and then proceeded to Tibet, where I spent another month meditating. I returned to New Delhi, spent a few days with some friends, and took a flight to Paris, France, in December 1974, where I spread the yoga knowledge for four years.

MY LAST MEETING WITH BAPUJI KRIPALU

It was late fall in 1979. I took a few disciples from my established yoga ashram in Haiti on a yoga tour in various cities in the U.S. We went to Sumneytown in Pennsylvania, where the Kripalu Ashram of Yogi Amrit Desai was located. I was well-received by Yogi Desai, who always had some interest in my Kkundalini yoga practices. I was introduced to his disciples, and we had a highly-energized satsang session at the Ashram.

The next day Yogi Desai took me and my disciples to Bapuji's Kripalu bungalow, who was now in the U.S. Arriving at his quarters, I bowed down to present my respect to him. He smiled as usual and was glad to see me again after so many years. He received me and my disciples in private. He was still silent and inquired on his slate about my yoga progress, and my activities. I told him that I had established yoga centers in Europe and the Kripalu Ashram in Haiti. He told me that is good, but do not forget to prioritize your own sadhana until the final stage. He gave me copies of his new writing about yoga, and his latest spiritual message during this year of *guru purnima* (gurus's birthday) to share with my disciples. That was my last encounter with Bapuji Kripalu. He left the United States for his homeland in 1980, and shortly after passed into eternal Samadhi.

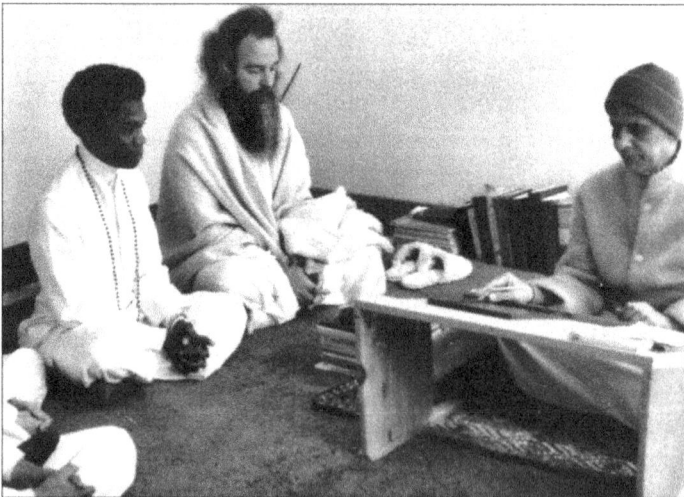

Dr. Lauture Massac (Yogi Darshan), Swami Yogeshwar, and Swami Kripalvananda (Bapuji) at Kripalu Ashram, Pennsylvania, 1979

CHAPTER III
WHAT IS HATHA YOGA?

LESSON 1   **PART 1**

The word *yoga* means *union*. The *hatha* has two syllables *Ha* and *Tha*. *Ha* means *sun*, *Tha* means *moon*. In a symbolic way, hatha yoga is the union of the sun and the moon. The sun symbolizes the flow of positive energy (Prana) within the human body, and the moon is the symbol for negative energy (Apana).

According to Oriental study of anatomy, these energies penetrate the entire body and vivify it. On that subject, research on Chinese acupuncture has shown a relationship in the manipulation of positive and negative energies in restoring physical equilibrium of health. (Xinnong, C. & Deng, L. 2000). On a higher level, hatha yoga permits the neutralization and mastery of those vital energies which allow the adept to enter more deeply into the sciences of meditation or raja yoga.

Hatha yoga is the way which leads us to universal consciousness. On a physical level, the adept of hatha yoga, who is called a hatha yogi, will draw from this equilibrium the different currents which animate the body, such as health, calmness, patience, nervous equilibrium, concentration, will power, and regenerative sleep.

PRELIMINARY RECOMMENDATIONS

Even though now-a-days yoga is quite popular in Western countries, when entering the realm of the holistic yoga, the neophyte is often confused. It may seem new, but it is so different from the Western lifestyle and thinking. And depending on your level of interest in yoga, it might surprise you at first. In a world filled with speed, commercialization, technology, and noise, you are trying to journey within yourself. Think of what it means: a break from old habits, and a beneficial break. During the short moment, too short, when you will find yourself in yoga, you should forget the noisy world around you. You will create a peaceful oasis where every day you can stop for a blessed moment.

We must draw your attention to this fact. You are about to enter into a very serious discipline. It is serious and somewhat hard for the common beginner. However, soon you will be rewarded. For more than five thousand years humans have been practicing yoga, but its necessity has never been more wanted and obvious as it is today.

All the material things and the electronic gadgets offered by modern civilization tend to alienate each one of us from the Self. We are solicited from all directions: the media, the TV commercials, the internet, the videos, the social network, and the more-and-more sophisticated mobile devices. We are constantly manipulated, and we feel that we are losing our self-identity. As a result, for the weak-minded, the nervous system breaks down more often, the heart gives up under stress, and the spine collapses. Physically and psychologically, what organism can resist such permanent nervous tension?

In this 21st century, as progress is replacing human values, the human race is moving toward its decadence. But still humans have at their disposal an accessible way to salvation. The wonderful discipline of yoga who was handed over to us by the great *rishis* (sages) of India, can keep us from falling. Yoga is for the whole being: the physical, the mental, and the spiritual. However, the one who believes only in the reality of the material world has also a chance to find his way through yoga. In the holistic yoga we are about to teach, you will find a great portion of it suitable to anyone who has an interest in yoga. We hope that it will bring to you, as it did to us, health, vitality, psychological wellbeing, spiritual fulfillment, and happiness.

THE DIFFERENCE BETWEEN
GYMNASTICS AND HATHA YOGA

Hatha yoga is the opposite of gymnastics, which is a sportive physical education. This basic notion must be accepted and understood from the very beginning. Gymnastics is a challenging sport. It is, first of all, movements, muscular work, spending of energy, and often fatigue. Hatha yoga is immobility, relaxation, energy build-up, endurance, and resting of the organs. Studies show that girls who are practicing gymnastics are vulnerable to delayed puberty, and both boys and girls are susceptible to stunted growth, due to extreme stress on the muscles (Ryan, J. 1995, 2000). It causes them to go through a certain number of contractions which require a lot of effort and bring about a loss of nervous energy in the body (Hardwood, R. et al., 2008).

Yoga acts upon the articulations, the ligaments, and the tendons to help to maintain or to restore elasticity. In hatha yoga, a posture is assumed and is maintained as long as possible without moving. Slowness of the movements and relaxation are the characteristics of hatha yoga.

Although a gentle, well-designed cardio workout program is believed to be beneficial for the heart, extreme gymnastics exercises make the heart do extra work, while yoga on the contrary provides rest. Gymnastics brings about an acceleration of the respiratory rhythm; yoga slows down the breathing. Gymnastics makes certain individuals feel tired; yoga always adds to all an excess of physiological wellbeing. Those essential differences show how opposed to each other those two disciplines are. Besides, yoga is not only teaching postures, or *asanas*; proper respiratory exercises constitute its major aspect.

CONCLUSION: In yoga, the movements are performed slowly. One gets into the posture slowly, keeps it for a certain length of time, and returns slowly to the starting point. There is no need for competition, haste, or useless spending of energy. Remember that in yoga, slowness is the key. If you intend to jump the steps of yoga, it is better for your health just to forget about it.

REQUIRED ATTITUDES IN YOGA

First is the will power. Although the discipline of yoga is a factor in strengthening the will power, one must have some of it to progress toward the goal.

The second requirement is patience. Haste and restlessness are the enemies of the Yogi. The student must realize that tomorrow, in three months, or within one year, he or she will definitely be able to assume the posture. One must not hurry, in order to avoid damaging a ligament. You need to think that you have the entire life ahead. If you are practicing yoga in a studio with other students, keep in mind that a competitive spirit has no place in yoga.

The third requirement is perseverance. Always learn to keep trying. Failure should not discourage you and cause you to give up. Progress will come in time, whatever your age, and whatever the amount of stiffness in your joints, spine, and articulations.

FAVORABLE MOMENT TO PRACTICE

The best moments to practice yoga are in the morning upon waking, and at night before dinner. However, due to busy schedule, not everyone might be able to keep such schedule; therefore, any time away from a heavy meal is good. For best result, the session should take place two to three hours after a meal. If you feel tired, don't skip your session. On the contrary, you will draw new energy and feel relief after a yoga workout.

THE PLACE TO PRACTICE

Now-a-days, modern yoga students are able to find a studio close by to practice yoga in a group. It is an ideal place to start, due to the camaraderie with other students. However, for advanced sadhakas who have made yoga a part of their lifestyle, they should pick a room with plenty of ventilations and away from noises, where they can be quiet and undisturbed. It is better to always use the same room, avoid smoking and entertaining too many guests who are not part of your lifestyle. If it is convenient to you, burn incense to attract positive vibrations. In the country, if the weather permits, you can practice outside, but keep away from curious stares. If you are physically able to exercise on the floor, use a yoga mat, a carpet, or a thick blanket.

For the sadhaka who wants to practice meditation alone, keep the room filled with positive vibrations and it should be considered as a sanctuary to you. If you are lucky enough to find a yoga center or ashram where regular satsangs are being conducted under a master, take advantage of such setting. Before a meditation session, always start first with yoga exercises. During your yoga practices, try not to be aware of the clock. If you don't have much time, do only a few postures follow by a few minutes of meditation. Never strain yourself or rush. Use some of your leisure time to practice yoga, but never use time that should be reserved for sleep.

THE DIRECTIVES FOR POSTURES
AND THE SCIENCE OF BREATHING (Pranayama)

For the postures and the breathing exercises (pranayama), read carefully the description of each exercise. You must be able to coordinate each description with the execution of the exercise. Read them again if necessary. Every time you are not sure about something, go back to the description and try again. Even when you think that you are doing a posture perfectly well, if you read again the description, you might find that you missed some details. Sometimes, many students feel that they have mastered a posture, when they later realized there is still improvement to be made. In fact, the body will tell you when you have mastered a yoga posture. Once you feel comfortable in it, with no strain on the muscles or ligament, then you can feel satisfied.

IMPORTANT ADVICE

Let your yoga session be a kind of communion with yourself and the cosmic energy. The real yoga is the science of reintegration. It puts us back into our own cosmic contact. *Yoga* means *to join*; it is a discipline which (when practiced in the right state of mind) links us to the universe in which we live and without which we could never exist. We should not forget that we bathe in the cosmic world of which our planet is an holistic part. That is why the yogi sees the cosmic world in the form of air, water, nourishment, and light which give life to all creatures.

Furthermore, the yoga session requires concentration, and almost a religious state of mind or communion. Only under those conditions can it be fully beneficial. There has to be a special inclination of the spirit and the body. Just like an opening-up of the entire being to the cosmic forces, it seeks to receive. In this perfect harmony, the yogi expresses gratitude towards the source of life it depends on.

ೞ

LESSON 1   PART 2
THE HATHA YOGA POSTURES
OM (The Maha-Mantra)

Before each yoga session, we sing OM (pronounced **aum**), which is the sacred Sanskrit monosyllable sound symbolizing the universal creation. By singing this cosmic sound, the individual reaches harmony within the self and the cosmic forces around. We also intone another Sanskrit word, *shanti*, which means *peace*. The sacred symbol OM creates a psychological and physiological effect as well as a highly spiritual influence. In yoga the sadhaka is not seeking only a self-peace, but also a peaceful state for all. That is why, before each yoga session or meditation, the sadhaka has to show humility, respect, and compassion towards all to be in perfect harmony with the cosmic.

The sound OM vibrates in the thoracic cage and stimulates the work of internal organs. It also vibrates in the neck, the head, and stimulates the glands responsible for basic hormonal secretions such as the thyroid and the pituitary glands. Repetition of this sound improves health, promotes youth and dynamism.

PSYCHO-PHYSIOLOGICAL RELAXATION

In materialistic modern society, total relaxation of the body and the mind is difficult to achieve when dynamism is often confused with agitation. Nevertheless relaxation, which helps to control stress, is important to the health. It is the basis for successful hatha yoga practice. We know that relaxation is indispensable to maintain optimum health. However, it has become one of the greatest challenges for hard-working people. Different means have been utilized to help achieve this end. They go from the super-comfortable massaging chair and refreshing Jacuzzis to the tranquilizing pills. So far, no modern invention has surpassed or equaled the natural technique of yoga. We can say that yoga is an antidote for depression, anxiety, phobia, and drug addiction.

Muscular relaxation is natural in animals; however, in modern human beings it must be rediscovered. Modern civilization forces us to use too much nervous energies. The pace of life imposed on us is causing anxiety, and the ever-mounting noises all constitute permanent aggression against the organism. These stressors make the organism feeble and accelerate the aging process.

Those who are caught in the daily actions have difficulty to fully relax their muscles. Even during sleep, some people remain tense. Sometimes what could have been a restful period on the contrary brings extra fatigue to them. In my private practice as a psychologist, I have seen the devastating effects of stress and anxiety in the lives of my clients. Even with all the comforts of life and all their electronic gadgets, they are unable to find a moment of joy. Some people told me that watching TV or going out to movies stressed them more. We can say that those folks who are able to relax the muscles and to calm the mental activity are the lucky ones in our modern time.

THE RESTING POSTURE - CORPSE POSTURE (Shavasana)

Shavasana is the main relaxing posture of yoga. It is the first posture we will describe, and it is also called "the corpse posture," even though the body must not be rigid. Lying flat on the back, the body must simply be as still as a corpse in order to experience total relaxation. This is a basic posture. When you have mastered it to a great extent, you will use it during the yoga session after one or several difficult postures to rest and to revitalize the organism.

EXECUTION: Lay down flat on the back, straighten out the legs with the feet kept apart. The arms are placed alongside of the body with opened palms. The back of the head is resting on the mat. The body should be oriented north-south (head toward the north) to attract positive magnetic flow of cosmic energy.

Before starting, stretch out the limbs, the torso, and the neck like a cat. Then concentrate on each muscle, beginning with the head, ending at the feet, while relaxing, until you no longer feel the muscles of your body. If you can do that, you have achieved a real state of relaxation. But remember—at first, muscles usually do not get completely relaxed. It might take you some practice before achieving a full resting moment lying on the floor.

Usually the body retains a certain amount of muscular tension that you will learn to ease. A nervous person will have difficulties in doing that. One will have to do a few contractions in between the position in order to fully appreciate the relaxation that follows. Lie down on the back (*Shavasana*), breathe in slowly while bending your right arm towards your head until it touches almost the floor, straighten it out and hold your breath. Then exhale suddenly and let the arm fall near the shoulder, do the same exercise with the left arm.

RESULTS: It will help you to be conscious of different muscle groups, in order to localize tension points and get rid of them.

VARIANT: Lay down flat on your back, close the eyes, and try to relax the face muscles, the forehead, and do not tighten the teeth. Let your mouth take a half smile (the Buddha smile). Remain absolutely still.

If you are doing right the posture, then you should feel the weight or the heaviness of the body. You must have the feeling that your body has become so heavy that it is sinking into the floor. Keep breathing slowly and evenly. As much as possible, observe an attitude of mental detachment. Try to imagine yourself floating on a still lake, on a cloud, free from all bonds, perfectly happy, and bathing in the vital currents of our planet.

This posture tends to straighten out the spinal curve, since it exerts a pressure by gravity action. If you are suffering from an exaggerated curvature of the spine, you should slip a small cushion under the hips, until you can do without it comfortably. The posture is perfected when the entire back can relax completely on the floor.

The goal of the *Shavasana* posture is to bring a complete relaxation of the entire nervous system in order to succeed in the yoga practice. In the beginning, it might be a little bit difficult, but by regular practice it soon will be mastered.

VARIATION: You can move the feet apart about 50 centimeters and keep the arms away from the body. And then keep the hands half-closed and the palms up.

COMPLETE BREATHING

Breathing is essential to life. The baby as soon out of the mother's womb took the first breath, and later in life, when ready to die, took the last breath. One can live several days without eating, drinking, or even sleeping, but one cannot live more than a few minutes without breathing. However, very few people breathe correctly. Incorrect breathing leads to a diminution of vitality. In yoga one can learn how to breathe correctly through the nose and not through the mouth. When breathing through the nose, one is protected against catching unwanted germs by a natural filter in the nose. Regular pranayama exercise helps in the development of the lungs to regularize the breathing rhythm. It is written in yogic literature that one is born with a set number of inhalations and exhalations. Learning how to preserve the numbers of those inhalations and exhalation could prolong one's life.

Furthermore, incomplete breathing brings about incomplete oxygenation of the blood and inadequate elimination of waste gases. As a result, the organism slowly becomes intoxicated. These explanations show how indispensable total breathing is to health. It is in your interest to study it carefully and to practice it whenever you can. Also, total breathing enables one to capture *prana,* or the cosmic vital energy, and to distribute it throughout the cells of the body.

ABDOMINAL BREATHING:

In this kind of breathing, the diaphragm fulfills its function perfectly, and it is very important. You need to work upon developing it until fully mastered. First, sit in any comfortable posture and keep the spine erect. Place one hand flat on the stomach to keep track of its movement. Start by expelling all the air from the lungs. The abdomen should become concave for the diaphragm to rise up. Slowly start inhaling through both nostrils. The abdomen is now filled with air and starts to go upward. The diaphragm lowers itself and comes to rest on the abdominal mass. Check the movement with the hand. When the diaphragm goes down at its lower point, start exhaling, and then progressively contract the abdomen.

This movement is continued slowly and completely. The hand accompanies it during inhalation as well as exhalation. Doing abdominal breathing, the upper part of the torso should remain still. In case it expands itself, that means you are doing it wrong. You should at once block the upper rib cage with a belt under the armpits.

ADVANTAGES TO THIS BREATHING EXERCISE: It airs out the lower part of the lungs, it massages the liver, kidneys, colon, genital organs, and increases gaseous exchanges.

MIDDLE BREATHING: In this breathing, the abdomen remains still, so does the upper torso. Only the middle part of the ribs cage rises and falls rhythmically. In the beginning, place one hand on the abdomen to check out its stillness.

UPPER BREATHING: In this variant, the abdomen and the middle part of the rib cage remain motionless. The collarbone and the shoulders rise up and the air fills the upper part of the lungs. This breathing is mostly natural to many women. Using together all the three exercises descried, we should obtain a complete set of breathing.

COMPLETE BREATHING: Take any comfortable sitting posture, inhale and exhale through both nostrils. Breathe in, filling first the abdominal and then the rib cage, while raising the shoulders. When the lungs are completely filled up (but not in exaggeration), breathe out. After that, lower the shoulders, empty the rib cage, and finally hollow the stomach in. Hold it for a few seconds, exhale the air, and then breathe normally.

One thing to remember is that the complete breathing is accomplished by linking the three types of breathing rhythmically and continuously. They are abdominal, middle, and upper breathing. For best results, try to practice between ten and fifteen minutes every day.

THERAPEUTIC EFFECTS: Those types of breathing exercises improve the blood circulation, increase oxygenation of the blood, rest the heart, and supply the body with vital cosmic energy (prana).

WARMING UP EXERCISES (For sitting postures)
In the next lesson, you will learn the first sitting posture, which is helpful for the practice of breathing exercise, or pranayama. During those two weeks it would be useful to do warming-up exercises in order to acquire elasticity of the limbs to facilitate the execution of the comfortable posture called *Sukhasana*.

Although some students are naturally born with flexible joints and they may experience less difficulty to sit in *Sukhasana*, they still will benefit in warming up the joints before proceeding in the executions of the asanas. Other, less flexible students may take several months before they can be able to sit comfortably for some time. By the way, let me remind you that *Sukhasana* is the easiest sitting posture to master (since the legs are not crossed), which is essential for the practice of meditation.

EXECUTION 1: In the sitting position, straighten the legs out. Fold the left one at a 90-degree angle, placing the underside of your left foot against the right thigh. Keeping the spine erect with the help of your left hand, press your left knee and try to make it touch the ground. Afterward, switch over to the right leg and repeat 3 or 4 times this exercise. This will prepare you for the student posture.

EXECUTION 2: Proceed as mentioned above, but the left foot should rest on the top of the right thigh instead of resting against its internal surface. Press down the left knee in trying to make it touch the floor. Hold it for a while, and then switch to the other leg. This exercise is somewhat more difficult than the previous one, and usually takes some more time before you can be comfortable in it.

EXECUTION 3: Sit down with both legs bent and catch the feet. Keep the soles together and push inward. Hold the position as long as you can, and with the elbows try to push the thighs toward the floor to make contact. This exercise will prepare the legs for the *Goraksa* posture.

EXECUTION 4: Kneeling, sit on your heels and then try to relax the ankles so that the back of the feet become truly in the line with your legs. Keep the position as long as you can. This exercise will prepare you for the posture of the adept.

WARM –UP EXERCISE (For Inverted Postures)
These exercises are excellent for the abdominal wall, and they also prepare the body for the inverted posture described in this lesson.

EXECUTION: Lie down on your back. Keep the arms alongside the body, and then slowly lift up the right leg while breathing in. Keep the right leg up for about 3 seconds, and then slowly lower it down to the horizontal position while exhaling. Repeat 4 to 6 times the exercise, and then alternate to the other leg. Then finally keep both feet together and lift them up and down several times, and then take a rest. Follow the breathing while raising up and down the legs.

During the following weeks, you should exercise the body to daily take the full resting posture, *Shavasana*. After the warm-up exercises and the complete abdominal breathing exercises, always take rest in *Shavasana*. This will help you to start with the second lesson with a better-relaxed body.

THE STUDENT POSTURE

To accomplish this simple posture, start with the warm-up exercise.

EXECUTION: Sit with the right leg straight out and fold the left one toward the underside of the right thigh. The right thigh is touching the floor. Keep the spine erect and relax the hand on the knees. Remain in this position motionless as long as you can, and then reverse the position. While in each position, just follow the breathing.

MENTAL FOCUS: On the heart.

RESULTS: This exercise helps to achieve a motionless state. It is also excellent to control the nervous system, and it brings suppleness to the knees and the joints.

THE ADEPT POSTURE

From all the warm-up exercises described you have practiced, you should be now ready to perform the complete adept posture.

EXECUTION: Sit on the heels. Relax and keep the spine erect. The hands are resting on the thighs, and the palms opened and facing upward. Remain motionless in the position with closed eyes, and just follow the breathing. You will get the full benefit of this posture by remaining in it for a long time.

MENTAL FOCUS: On the heart center, or *Anahat Chakra.*

RESULTS: This posture is also one of the meditating postures. It prepares the student for the development of physical and mental balance, and helps in the control of the nervous system. This posture is excellent to strengthen the articulation of the ankles and the feet. It is also very helpful in the practice of pranayama and in the complete understanding of the science of breathing.

THE REVERSE POSTURE (Viparita-Karani)

The last warm-up exercises should have prepared you for this posture.

EXECUTION: Lie down on your back. Keep the feet together and place the legs straight, then lift them up slowly while inhaling. Continue the movement of the legs backward. With the help of the hands placed under the hips, raise your pelvis but do not jerk it. The legs and the thighs are straight at an angle of about 45 degrees and should try to touch the floor. The feet are now beyond the vertical plane of your head. You should find a point of balance where you are comfortable, and then take a deep and slow abdominal breath. In remaining in this posture, the thyroid gland is being affected by the pressure of your chin on the throat. At first, you may feel a slight discomfort, but it should go away after a while. Remain in the position as long as you can without feeling much discomfort, while breathing normally. Finally, get back to the initial position and take rest in *Shavasana*.

THERAPEUTIC RESULTS: It is an excellent posture for blood circulation in the legs. It is restful for the heart, strengthens the thyroid gland, tones the facial skin and muscles, and may prevent wrinkles.

BREATHING: It should be very deep and slow. While in this posture, contracting the abdominal and the anus muscles will help in the evacuation of gas.

THE TREE POSTURE (Ardha-Vriksasana)

EXECUTION: Standing up, keep the arms alongside the body. Lift up the left leg, and try not to bend much the knee. Place the left instep against the convex part of the right knee, where the left foot can find support. Try to find your balance while standing on the right foot. Remember that your left foot is pressing against the right knee. The left leg has to remain in the plane of the body. Keep the arm relaxed, while trying to find your balance. After some time, give up the position and alternate to the other leg. The breathing should be normal, and you should concentrate on your balance.

THERAPEUTIC EFFECTS: It tranquilizes the nervous system. It helps to develop a sense of balance and self-control.

MOVEMENTS FOR THE NECK

Now we will study some neck movements, which you can practice often to get relief from neck stiffness. We will also practice some eye rotations to maintain healthy vision.

As part of warm-up exercises before a full hatha yoga session, take a comfortable sitting position and perform the following movements:

FLEXION: Lower your head forward until the chin touches the chest. Press the chin down for a few seconds, and then raise up slowly the head.

EXTENSION: Slowly let the head fall backward, and then press it back as much as you can while focusing for a few seconds on stress relief of the neck, then bring the head back slowly to the initial position.

ROTATION: Turn the head to the right as far as it will go. The movement must be very slow. Hold it a few seconds and then slowly come back to the starting point. Repeat the rotation several times on one side, and reverse to the other side.

LATERAL INCLINATION: Starting from an upright position, incline your head to the right without turning it. Go as far as possible, and then hold it for a few seconds before returning to the starting position. Do the same action inclining to the left. Repeat the movement several times on both sides and then relax.

EYE MOVEMENTS

FOCUSING BETWEEN THE EYEBROWS: The student takes a sitting position. The breathing is regular, and the eyes are kept wide open. Turn your eyes toward the point between the eyebrows. If you feel a strain, breathe deeply, and close the eyes and start over again after resting the eyes.

FOCUS ON THE NOSE: The concentration should be on the tip of the nose.

LATERAL MOVEMENT OF THE EYES: From the same sitting posture, while breathing normally, stare at a point straight ahead of you. Then direct your gaze to the right as far as possible. Hold on to the position and bring the eyes back to the neutral position. Start again the same movement to the left. Repeat this exercise for about 3 to 5 times.

EYE ROTATIONS: From a sitting posture, while breathing slowly, look straight ahead, and then look up and make a circular motion with the eyes by looking down left, right, and then up again. Do a complete circle 3 times, and repeat the exercise from the opposite direction.

LESSON 1   **PART 3**
INTRODUCTION TO HIGHER YOGA

As you have already been told, the third part of every lesson will be reserved for HIGHER YOGA. The materialistically-minded students who practice yoga only for their physical benefits do not have to study this part except for a few chapters which we will indicate.

However, they should not think that yoga has also a spiritual path which they don't need and therefore disregard it. There are some moments in our life where hardships can cause our views of the world to change. For example, fatal illness or the sudden loss of a loved one. Serious ordeals in our lives can make us realize that existence is a hard school that can't be ignored. Every one of us at any given time can become suddenly conscious of the higher realities. No materialist is immune to that sudden illumination which is called "Grace," and which can transform your life. We hope the dark days of your life will soon be followed by sunshine and will bring light into your life.

THE BASIC GOALS

In this part devoted to higher yoga, we will bring the same scientific concern we had for the teaching of the physical yoga. Every day modern science is getting closer to the occult science; the space between them is getting smaller and smaller. The magic of communication is able to bring instantly a live happening event in any corner of the world to our living room. The continuous discoveries of new planets in the infinite cosmos have made science fiction a reality. The times are near when, according to this saying, "Things hidden will be revealed." We want to make it clear that the teaching we will now introduce is only a transitory outlook on truth. As we progress toward the eternal goal, our conception of truth changes. We go from one state of consciousness to another one that is refined and more inclusive. Each succeeding state of consciousness unveils a different truth which it contains, and which goes beyond previously acquired knowledge. That is why we say that yoga is a spiritual science. Just as in human science, always further explorations and research are needed.

Furthermore, we can say that each state of consciousness corresponds to a transitory truth. This is why even the greatest scientist must remain humble. None can claim to have penetrated even a significant percentage of the secret of the cosmos. Yoga cannot be understood in its essence nor can its effects be fully appreciated without certain knowledge of things. We will explain this in the third part of each lesson. We must not forget three centuries ago, (and what are three centuries in the story of evolution?) that Galileo was put on house arrest and condemned by the Catholic Church for "vehement suspicion of heresy" for declaring that the earth was turning around the sun (Bryant, W. 1918).

We do not have the pretention of bringing an intangible truth. We only hope to make clear certain essential notions which the average person of our times should become familiar with. Since the beginning of time, there has been the privilege of a few CHOSEN ONES who have carried through the ages the light of the world. These messengers have only been able to present the truth in a way acceptable to the people of their times. When this new era is dawning, humanity must take one more step on the way and accede to a greater understanding of truth.

VISIBLE AND INVISIBLE HUMAN BEING

The real yoga is the science of the holistic human being—physical, mental, and spiritual. We will make an attempt to define and explain what is meant by holistic human being.

For the materialist, a human being is only physical and mental. No one discusses the existence of the aspects. The physiological yoga which we will teach in the second part of our lessons is dedicated to this subject. Even though human beings are mortals and will return to ashes, some believe only in themselves. They believe in the world which is revealed by their senses. Being materialistic is the characteristic of modern science. At the same time, hasn't it opened to us an invisible world as tangible and as great as the world we comprehend through the senses?

In its attempts to penetrate the secrets of matter, 21st century science has reached the border of the occult. With constant discoveries of faraway planets in other galaxies, scientists will soon be ready to reveal the last secret. The last step will be cleared when they will admit that energies are not blind, but intelligent, and the difference between spirit and matter is a question of degrees of vibration.

Light, sound, color, and other sensations reveal the world to us. Quantum science now accepts the idea that the universe is made of energies and vibrations (Folger, 2001). But how limited is the sphere offered to our perception? We are only partially conscious of all manifestations of the Universe. The realm of infra-red, ultra-violet rays, and ultra-sonic is beyond our perception. They make up another universe as real and which may be much vaster than the one we are familiar with, but so different that we cannot imagine it. If we were sensitive to all of those vibrations, the hidden and marvelous aspect of our universe would have been revealed to us.

No doubt, as the yogic scriptures revealed, there is another form of energy (prana) subtler than those we have just mentioned. Science will discover it one day as it discovered rays and wave-lengths. The fact that prana remains a part of yogic self-discovery does not mean that it does not exist.

The part of the universe we can perceive is only a small part of the whole. Therefore, it is the same for the ordinary person to whom only the grossest appearance is perceived to our senses. Only the material aspect of us is visible, although we would be nothing without the multiple energies that animate us. If those vital energies escape, we soon become nothing but dust. What is the origin of these energies which animate the body? Do they disappear with it or do they go back to some cosmic source? Is the transitory shell of the body the sole component of us? Or do we sometimes become aware of a subtle body, the one which is not revealed to our physical senses?

We have been asking those questions since the beginning of time. Some light has shed into our brain; an inner voice has told us that this body is not our own reality. We have to discover ourselves and to seek for eternal life through the labyrinth of perishable matter. Yoga has become a guide in this search. The science of the holistic person—this is the yoga we are teaching. Physical (hatha) yoga is for the body, and it is necessary. The body has to be treated well, for it is the most precious instrument which will enable us to reach a HIGHER REALITY. The organism must be healthy and function perfectly. Spiritual fulfillment can only be reached if the body is in perfect health and under control. If we are preoccupied all the time with treating a body which is sick, then how can we hear the voice of our Spirit?

It is through matter that the Spirit is revealed. This search is the highest stage in yoga. In as much as the postures and the breathing techniques help to develop mastery over the body, other techniques permit us to make contact with the invisible part of us. Overall, those methods promote the illumination of the material being through the absorption of subtle energies.

Finally, like physical yoga, spiritual yoga also demands discipline. A consistent effort of the sadhaka is needed. One has to reorient one's life and give up many false satisfactions on the material level. One has to give away some of the surplus of the need and some of the desires in order to reach the goal. Finally, at the end of this road, the eternal truth is awaiting the sadhaka, and good health, peace, and happiness will be within the reach.

CHAPTER IV

MENTAL CONCENTRATION

This lesson will deal more directly with the postures and the science of breathing (pranayama), which will constitute the second part. In order for those two techniques to be fully beneficial, they must be complemented by a study of MENTAL CONCENTRATION, especially in the case of the science of breathing. The goal of this concentration is to strengthen the mental by the physiological influence of the physical exercises.

It is not necessary to explain how the state of mind influences the body. Note, however, that in modern psychology, the mind-body connection is well-established. Thousand years ago, the wise rishis who discovered the science of yoga already knew this fact. That is why they have used the mental component in order to increase the beneficial effects of hatha yoga. By directing our thoughts to any particular point of the body, we provoke an accumulation of energy there. That is why many methods of physical education have obtained better results by coupling the mental concentration with physical work.

In yoga, mental activity must accompany the posture, as well as in breathing exercises.

While executing a posture, mental concentration must be focused on the correct execution of the movement performed by the limbs. The breathing must be controlled.

In the science of breathing, or pranayama, since the concentration is not directed on any posture, it must be focused on the respiratory rhythm cadence, and on the vital energy (prana), which flows into the organism.

While holding your breath, you should also imagine the vital energy entering all the organs of the body, including the endocrine gland and the nervous system. It takes much effort to attain a steady mental concentration. You should try to forget about exterior stimuli, worries, or the passing of time, and focus all your attention on the posture or the breathing you are working on. If you allow any negative thoughts to enter your mind, these will generate a succession of other thoughts, and you cannot keep a proper degree of concentration.

Mental wandering is the characteristic of an entrained ordinary mind. The human mind is continuously invaded by thoughts bearing no connection with one another. Those thoughts seem to come and go as they please, just like rabbits. Such uncontrolled thoughts really agitate the mind and make it very crowded. First you must stop this movement, then focus your attention on one point and try to hold it there by using your willpower. In the beginning for some sadhakas it is difficult to stop the flow of the thoughts, but with regular training, after some time, surely a good result will come out of it.

Yogic experience shows that it is better to practice those exercises in a quiet place and at a time when you are not in a hurry. It is recommended to keep the eyes closed for better concentration. This technique is favorable for mental counting of holding time of the breath while focusing on the heart chakra. After a few months of practice, you should feel heat irradiating the heart region when your breathing exercises are accompanied by concentration. It is the manifestation of prana. The practice of mental concentration will not only increase the benefits of the postures and the breathing exercises, it will also get you into the habit of ordering your thoughts, which will help you to better solve your problems with a clearer outlook on life.

Mental concentration opens the door to higher deeds. It is a stairway from which you can get access to the higher levels of yoga. More details on the actual practice of mental concentration and its effects on spiritual life will be available in part 3 of the third lesson. Now you will practice mental concentration by doing the following exercises. It is an excellent concentration exercise. It will enable you progressively to control your cerebral activities. You should become familiar with your own cardiac rhythm by counting your pulse rate. By doing so, your thoughts will be occupied on this work only, and no foreign thoughts will be able to disturb your concentration. Such concentration will allow you to make faster progress, and it is easier to do than to concentrate on a particular spot of the body.

Those who have difficulties in concentrating at the beginning should use this method for a longer period of time. For more details on concentration, see part 3 of the next lesson. For the time being, here are three exercises for concentration.

EXERCISE 1: VISUAL CONCENTRATION ON THE TIP OF THE NOSE

Take any comfortable posture, focus your eyes on the tip of the nose, hold on as much as you can, thinking of nothing else except on the need to stay motionless. Breathe slowly and normally.

EXERCISE 2: MENTAL CONCENTRATION BETWEEN THE EYEBROWS

From any comfortable sitting posture, close the eyes and imagine a shiny point between your eyebrows. Concentrate on this point, think of nothing else, and breathe slowly. This exercise will introduce you to meditation.

EXERCISE 3: CONCENTRATION ON THE HEART CHAKRA

You can either take a sitting posture or the resting one (*Shavasana*). Try to be conscious of your heart beats. In a quiet place, concentrate on your cardiac rhythm. After a certain period of time, you should be able to feel the beatings of your heart in your chest.

ELEMENTARY NOTION ABOUT PRANA

It is quite impossible to learn the holistic yoga without knowing something about prana, the planetary cosmic energy which, through yoga, a sadhaka can learn to collect and utilize in the body.

In the first lesson, we said that the yogi must practice the exercise and the posture through mental concentration in order to get in touch with prana. In the third part of our studies, we will study prana in detail and the way in which it is received and distributed. However, it is good to know about it as early as possible, and to be aware of the fact that the major effects of yoga result from prana, this subtle electro-magnetic energy.

Prana brings health, nervous equilibrium, and vitality to the entire being. Perhaps you might be skeptical about its reality. However, through regular practice of concentration and breathing exercises, you will feel warm rays spreading through your whole body. Then you will no longer doubt of its reality.

ﾞ

LESSON 2   PART 2
HATHA YOGA POSTURES, OR ASANAS

We hope that during those past two weeks you have become familiar with the preliminary warm-up exercises and the first asanas. You can continue to practice them every day until your hips, knees, and ankles become quite comfortably supple.

On the other hand, by now you must be thoroughly familiar with the posture of COMPLETE RELAXATION (*Shavasana*), and quite advanced with deep breathing exercises. You should continue to practice them for the next fifteen days along with some other asanas and breathing exercises you will learn in this lesson. In order to keep the body fit, you should always maintain each exercise or series of exercises to unwind the body and bring complete rest to it.

SURYA-NAMASKAR (Salutation to The Sun)

Now we are going to learn one of the most important postures in hatha yoga:

THE SURYA-NAMASKAR –This posture, if it is performed slowly in the right way along with the correct breathing, will bring suppleness and full energy to the whole body. This posture makes all the parts of the body work. Sometimes, if you do not have much time to practice yoga in the morning, do only the Surya-Namaskar three times and then rest for five minutes. This is sufficient to keep you fit for the whole day. It is a complete set of postures in the whole hatha yoga system.

The Surya-Namaskar is divided into twelve movements or postures, beginning from the starting point. In the beginning, you do not have to execute them as they are perfectly performed on some photos. You do as you can, and one day perfection will automatically come. In fact, the Surya-Namaskar prepares the whole body for a better performance of other asanas.

Traditionally, before starting with any asana, the yogis always start with Surya-Namaskar.

EXECUTION:

1) Standing up, facing east or north, keep the feet joined to each other. The hands are folded at the chest level. Follow your breathing and concentrate on it for a while.

2- Bend your bust backward as far as possible. Bring the arms up while inhaling slowly and retain the air.

3- Come down while holding on to the breath.

4- Straighten up the left leg behind, inhale, with both hands on the floor.

5- Straighten up the right leg behind and hold on the breath.

6- Bring the whole body down while exhaling. Keep the forehead, chest, and knees on the floor.

7- Hands on the floor, the legs straight down and flat on the floor, bring the bust up while inhaling.

8- Keep the hands and feet at their initial position, and bring the body upward, head down and keep holding the breath.

9- Bring the left leg toward your hands while exhaling.

10- Bring the right leg toward your hands. Keep the breathing and stand up, head down with the arms touching the feet.

11- Come up again and bend the bust backward as far as possible while inhaling.

12- Come back again from the starting point, both hands folded at the chest level, and keep breathing normally.

SUKHASANA (Comfortable Posture)

This is the first sitting posture we will describe. It is used mostly for meditation, breathing exercises or pranayama. It is a preparation for the perfect posture (*Siddhasana*). If you have done all the preliminary warm-up exercises in the first lesson, you will have a better chance to succeed in it. If you cannot do it right away, do not get discouraged. Keep on practicing the warm-up exercises and try to do the posture every day. It might take several months to perform it.

EXECUTION: Sit down, fold the right leg and place the right ankle in front of the perineum; then fold your left leg and with the help of your right hand, place it on top of your bent right leg. The knees should be on the floor or as close as possible. Keep the spine erect, the hands should be relaxed on the knees.

CONCENTRATION: On the heart center.

BREATHING: It should be done deeply and slowly. Try to remain in the posture as long as possible. Afterward, spread out the legs and relax.

It will depend on the suppleness of your hips, knees, and ankles. In the beginning you may feel uncomfortable, and the posture might be a little painful to you. It is a good way to prepare you for more advanced postures. Keep on trying and do it every day, but do not force the limbs.

RESULTS: It gives nervous equilibrium, suppleness of the articulations of the legs and feet, favorable posture to perform pranayama and to sit for meditation.

PAVANA MUKTASANA (Wind liberation posture)

EXECUTION: Sit down with folded legs, with the feet flat on the floor, and keep the heels as close as possible to the buttocks. Extend the arms behind your back and put the hands flat on the floor. Keep the spine erect. Take a deep breath in, and slowly try to rest your forehead on your knees, while breathing out. There will be a pressure on the pectoral muscle, which is attached to the ribs and sternum. Keep the posture, hold on the breath, lift up the bust while breathing in, and then breathe out. Repeat this exercise three to four times, and then relax.

The farther the arms are from the body, the harder the posture is. If you feel a little pain around your ribs, ease the tension and it will diminish.

CONCENTRATION: It should be upon the heart and the throat center.

RESULTS: A powerful workout is taking place on the pectoral muscle, suppleness of the spine, and the pose has a beneficial effect on the throat, tonsils, the thyroid glands, and the thymus. Try as much as possible to keep the knees together and bring the heels close to the buttocks.

GORAKSA-ASANA (Goraksa posture)

Review the third warm-up exercise in the first lesson, which is a preparation to this posture.

EXECUTION: Sit down with folded legs; place the toes to toes and the heels against each other. With both hands, catch the feet together and try to bring them toward the perineum. The knees should go down on the floor. Keep the arms straight, and the torso erect. For those who have stiff legs, this posture often takes a long time and some persistence to be mastered, although it is a basic posture.

BREATHING: Slowly and deeply.

CONCENTRATION: On the heart region.

Before doing this posture, it is better to practice other preliminary leg exercises and the third warm-up exercise in the first lesson. This asana is not a very easy one to master. You should keep on with the practice and never give it up. If we introduce it so early in the second lesson, it is because it increases tremendously suppleness of the hip joint. It is a preparation to the posture of meditation which should be learned as soon as possible.

VARIATION OF THE GORAKSA-ASANA:

From this posture, try to reach your toes with the forehead. Breathe in at first with the torso erect and lower your bust forward. Breathe out while pressing your thighs with your elbows. Rest the forehead on the toes if you can, lungs empty and holding your breath for a few seconds, then straighten the torso and bring the bust back up slowly while breathing in, and then breathe out again.

CONCENTRATION: Focus on the suppleness of the legs and on the heart.

RESULTS: It is one of the best postures to attain suppleness of the hips and joints. It prevents rheumatism of the hips and the legs.

ADVICE: As long as you have not mastered this posture, you should continue with the warm-up exercises of the first lesson. You may experience in the beginning a little discomfort in the joints, but after some time, it will vanish. Do not strain with the elbows. Exert the pressure very slowly, never jerk, and above all never give up the hope of attaining the posture in all its perfection.

THE HALF-COBRA (Ardha-Bhujanga Asana)
FIRST POSTURE
EXECUTION: Place the left foot flat on the floor; the left leg is bent. The right leg is extended behind as far as it will go. The arms alongside the body, the torso is erect. Exert a maximum pressure on the left leg, and then try to extend the right one as much as possible. Keep the torso erect and try to touch the floor with your fingers. Switch the legs and reverse the posture.

SECOND POSTURE: (Variant)
Place the left hand on the knee, the right hand and the arm straight alongside of the right thigh, and then rotate the head and the bust toward the right. Switch the legs and reverse the posture with the rotation.

BREATHING: Slow and normal.

CONCENTRATION: On the spinal column.

RESULTS: It promotes suppleness of the spine and will correct its deformations. Beneficial for the kidneys, the renal glands; strengthens the lymphatic system, promotes suppleness of the hip and the thigh muscles.

FOOT-STRETCH POSTURE (Uttanpadasana)
Lying on your back, keep the legs straight and lift them up to a 45-degree angle with the floor. The arms are straight and held parallel to the legs. Hold on to this position while breathing slowly, and then very slowly lower the legs, the torso, and come back to the initial position, and then relax in *Shavasana* posture.

BREATHING: Slowly and deeply.
CONCENTRATION: On the abdomen.
RESULTS: It is an excellent tonic for the muscles. It prevents grease and dropsy in the belly and strengthens the abdominal wall.

POSTERIOR-STRETCH POSTURE (Pascimottanasana)

This is a basic posture. You should study it carefully. It acts upon the back muscles, which it stretches along with the abdominal muscles, which cause it to contract. There are two postures within it, a preliminary one and a complete one.

PRELIMINARY POSTURE: While sitting in a comfortable position, stretch your arms back, the hands flat on the floor. Expel the air from the lungs and breathe in deeply. Slowly lower the torso forward while exhaling and bring the head closer to the knees. Try to touch the knees if possible with the forehead. Your hands will move slightly and come closer to the body.

If you do not succeed right away, keep on trying to lower slowly your torso more and more. Never proceed suddenly, and keep on resting your head on the knees for a few seconds, empty the lungs, and raise yourself up while breathing in.

BREATHING: Follow the breathing procedure described above.
CONCENTRATION: On the solar plexus.

COMPLETE BASIC POSTURE OF PASCIMOTTANASANA

Lie down on your back with feet together, breathe in deeply, and raise the trunk up slowly by using the power of the abdominal muscles. Bend it forward slowly, grab the ankles with both hands and expel the air from the lungs. By pulling on your ankles, you cause the torso to lean farther forward and your head to reach the knees. At this point, the elbows should touch the ground and the knees should not be bent. Hold on to the position for a while, and then raise yourself slowly while breathing in, and breathe out. Repeat the posture three or four times and then take rest in *Shavasana* position.

TWO ADVICES:

1-If you cannot arrive at a sitting position from the prone position by abdominal contraction, start the posture from the sitting position or while lying down. Help yourself with the elbows and the hands.

2-If you cannot get your head close to the knees without bending them and feel a little pain at the back of your thighs, it is due to the muscles at the back of your thighs, which are stiff. Eventually, by regular practice, they will loosen away along with the dorsal muscles.

RESPIRATORY RHYTHM: Let us remind you of this: Breathe in before raising the torso, breathe out while bending toward the knees. Hold on the breath while keeping the position, breathe in again while raising yourself up, and then exhale while going back down. If you want to keep the posture for a longer length of time, breathe superficially while doing so.

CONCENTRATION: On the solar plexus.

THERAPEUTIC RESULTS: It loosens the spine and the posterior muscles of the thigh, strengthens the abdominals, and reduces sciatic muscle disorders. It rejuvenates the lymphatic system, and it is excellent for the prostate gland, the sexual glands, and the pancreas.

PRANAYAMA

We hope that in the past two weeks you have come to assimilate properly the abdominal breathing exercises (abdominal, middle, and higher respiration), and that you are also practicing the complete deep breathings regularly. If not, you should keep on practicing them.

Now here are some basic notions which will help you to understand the science of breathing. Please study them carefully and always keep them in mind. Breathing renews the supply of the oxygen carried by the blood and flushes the gaseous waste from the organism. Later on, in other lessons, we will dwell more intensively upon the physiological effects of the blood circulation and we will establish their relationship to yoga.

The yogis say that through breathing exercises, they can capture along with the oxygen the prana which is distributed to all cells of the organism and which brings them new vitality. They say that the prana is the earth's vital energy, which comes from the sun. Thus we can understand the importance of retaining the breath in the practice of pranayama. During the retention, the prana spreads itself throughout the body in all the nervous system and the glands. It is distributed in the cells of the body through the media of the blood and the neurons in the brain. You will notice through personal experiences that the statement of the yogis is correct, but it might take you several months or years to realize it. You will also notice that the natural automatic way of breathing can also be controlled at will. By acting willfully upon the rhythm of their respiratory system, the yogis can control not only their heartbeats, but almost the entire organic system.

However, your ambition should be more humble than that. You should seek to let prana do its work naturally and automatically in the body, in order to achieve balanced mind and good health. We know that anger and fear generate an emotional state of mind which reacts upon the respiratory system. They start a physiological change in the body by provoking some internal secretion inside it. However, the process can be reversed by changing the respiratory rhythm, and then it becomes possible to dominate the emotion. Therefore, the sadhaka who practices regularly pranayama can attain a great nervous equilibrium and the control of temperament and tendencies.

If we agree that the frequent emotional reactions caused by the aggravations of modern life are responsible for many physiological disorders, then we can say that the human who has the knowledge to dominate them has a better chance to remain in good health. The science of pranayama offers to the practitioner the means to do so.

However, we have to warn the sadhaka about too much of exultation if the complete breathing can be practiced without any danger. The retention of the breath, or *kumbhaka pranayama*, could have some risks. You should observe the rules and proceed carefully, usually under the guidance of an accomplished master.

In the beginning, the retention should be short, and the length of time should be increased as the organism is getting used to it. Those who are suffering from heart diseases, blood pressure, or other respiratory disorders should avoid practicing such type of pranayama. You should notice that certain types of pranayama should not be practiced without proper diet.

PRANAYAMA: THE RHYTHMIC BREATHING

Take any comfortable posture of your choice. First, exhale completely to empty the lungs, then take a deep breath (inhale), and then very slowly exhale the air through both nostrils regularly. Repeat this exercise seven to ten times and then take a rest.

CONCENTRATION: The focus should be on the audible sound of the coming and going of the air.

KUMBAKA NO. 1(Retention)

SECOND PRANAYAMA: Sit in a comfortable posture. First exhale completely, and then inhale slowly through the right nostril, stop the breath as long as you can, and then exhale through the same nostril. Inhale through the left nostril, hold on to the air as long as you can, and then exhale through the same one. Repeat three to six times in each nostril, and then breathe normally.

CONCENTRATION: While retaining the breath, imagine that the prana is spreading in all the nervous system, and is bringing to you comfort and health.

KUMBHAKA NO. 2

Sit in a comfortable position, take a deep breath, and then exhale to empty the lungs. Soon after, take another deep breath and close both nostrils and stop your breath as long as possible without exaggerating (a few seconds), and then exhale. Repeat it three to six times and then breathe normally.

CONCENTRATION: It is upon the heart region.

LESSON 2 PART 3

HIGHER YOGA
The Discovery of the Inner Spiritual Being

If you have decided to go towards the discovery of your inner spiritual being, you should know that it is only from the physical body that the way is open and not through the intellect alone. In the holistic yoga, the body is considered as the laboratory in which esoteric spiritual discovery is explored.

The duty of the one who is progressing towards the spiritual light is to maintain the body in perfect physical condition as far as it is possible. It is the tool and a means which will enable you to perform proper spiritual work. If the tool is not up-to-date, the workman will not be able to do a good job.

This body that the false prophets have cursed should be the object of your best care. Its health should remain in good condition. Except for some cases, usually an advanced yogi should not suffer from any chronic diseases. Or we can put it this way: the disease of a yogi is not the same as the disease of an ordinary person. If a yogi is attacked by any passing infection, she has the knowledge to deal with it. Usually it will not last long, and its effect on the general health will be minimal. A yogi is a source of light, and the light disperses diseases which are of a gloomy origin.

By practicing regularly hatha yoga, your health will be maintained. It will help you to keep the body in a condition in which you will feel the peaceful and perfect working condition of the organs. However, one thing you should also never forget is that the body should be your servant and not your master. Its needs, its desires, its reactions should be under your control. The yogi remains the sovereign master of his body. For that, you should regularize your life by living a temperate life. It is the base of the superior yoga.

To succeed in the first step, you should be able to master the physical body, to dominate your emotions and desires. It is toward this goal that hatha yoga and pranayama will lead you. However, you should also control your sexual desires. It is very important for full success in the practice of higher yoga. It is the key which will open the door to salvation (if it is your goal!).

In order for the body not to remain anymore an obstacle to the Spirit, it should be not only controlled, but purified. Through the regular check-up of sexual desires, this process can be achieved. You should also follow a proper diet, convenient to your own metabolism. Your body should not be like a garbage can, in which you throw everything and at any time. The habit of eating all the time should also be controlled.

Alcoholism and smoking bring toxins not only to the physical body, but they kill the searching possibilities of the mind to discover its real self. The yogic moral rules (Yama-Niyama) should be put into practice. Make non-violence a major rule in your life. You should restrain yourself in causing any trouble or pain to anyone. The hatred which is virtual in your heart, as soon as it shows itself out, should at once be chased away. For that, one should concentrate on positive thoughts only. In that way, you are putting at your disposal the polarity law of nature.

Ego, jealousy, hatred, lust, and greed should be replaced by modesty, fraternity, love, purity, and self-content. Truth should be your guide. You should always try to maintain it even at any cost. You should always try to show a permanent good humor. A sad person could never be a yogi or a messenger of light. Enjoy all the good things in life at your disposal. However, be non-attached to people or to material things. This is the main rule to any higher spiritual progress. Only the eternal Spirit should be the real focus of your life. The advanced yogi remains unmoved and unaffected by whatever troubles are going on in the world, as they are so common these days. Those troubling upheavals are necessary for the evolution of humans, so you should not be affected. But you should not only retain yourself, you should also give and help whenever you have a chance to do so, without expecting any fruit of your action or anything in return. In thought, speech, and action, you should manifest the virtue of love—not ordinary selfish love, as most people are talking about. It should not be the love dedicated to one person or one's family, but to the whole world creation. Such a love is not a sporadic emotional affection, it is real life. Just like the sun which is spreading its rays upon all creatures, it is impersonal towards the good and the bad.

If you try to practice those advices of higher yoga, you will enjoy soon the unexpected fruits of them. Slowly, slowly your body will be purified and will become lighter. The good cosmic vibrations will spread all over your being. Your physical body and your mind will no longer be obstacles to the dawning of the spiritual light. You will feel that it is easier to lift up yourself to the Supreme Spirit, to be in permanent contact and communion with higher energies, and ever nearer to the kingdom of God.

CHAPTER V

THE POSTURES (ASANAS)

Before starting with this lesson, you should review all the preceding ones, which we have already studied. You must persist, particularly on the *Goraksasana*, which might take you a long time to master. Persist also on *Shavasana*, the complete resting posture of the first lesson.

Here are some more practical advices about *Shavasana*. In this resting posture, take the habit of breathing very slowly. Always try mentally to control your heart rhythm, which should slow down. Always try to relax all your muscles for a complete détente. Keep trying to empty your mind with all thoughts in order to concentrate on the inner self, which is peace and void. At least try to keep yourself in harmonious tune with the cosmic vibrations. In this way, your conscious will be in touch with the superconscious field, and all the cosmic energies you desire will come to you.

Slowly, slowly peace, calmness, détente, and self-confidence, which are the characteristics of the cosmic forces, will spread in you and will be established. However, this will not happen in one day; you have to persevere for some time.

FIRST POSTURE: VRIKSHASANA (Tree posture)
EXECUTION: Standing up, join the feet with the arms along the body, lift up the right foot and catch it with both hands, and let it rest tightly on your left thigh. To keep your balance, bend your body a little bit to the left while executing the posture, and then after, straighten it up, bringing both hands folded to your chest. You should try to keep your balance on your left leg without shaking. In the beginning you may find it difficult to keep your balance. If there is anything nearby, such as a wall or a table, hang on to it. After some time, you should be able to stand perfectly well on your own, on one leg without shaking. When you are able to execute the posture, keep it as long as possible, and after that reverse the position. You can also do a variant with the arms, by relaxing them alongside

the body, thumbs of the hands bending and touching the index. Repeat this posture three times on each leg.

RESPIRATORY RHYTHM: It should be slow and complete.

MENTAL CONCENTRATION: First on the psychic and physical equilibrium, and then on the heart center (Anahat chakra).

SECOND TREE POSTURE (Vriksasana Variant)

This variant, which is more advanced than the first one, consists of changing the position of the feet, which should rest upon the thigh. For that, the joints of the knees should be quite supple.

EXECUTION: Starting as described before, place the right leg (the ankle resting upon the left thigh) below the hip. The heel should be facing upward. Place your hands folded near the chest and maintain the position as long as possible.

RESPIRATORY RHYTHM: Same as the first one.

CONCENTRATION: Also the same.

THERAPEUTIC RESULTS OF THESE TWO POSTURES: They are classified among the postures for physical and mental balance. They produce a powerful beneficial effect upon the nervous equilibrium and help to develop concentration. The second one also brings suppleness to the joints of the knees and ankles, and will prepare the legs for *Padmasana* (the lotus posture).

You should keep improving the *Sukhasana* (comfortable posture). During the past two weeks, if you are able to perform properly the *Sukhasana*, you should be happy. If not, keep on with the warm-up exercises which will bring more suppleness to the joints, and keep on trying it regularly. Some students will take several months before they can accomplish the *Sukhasana* posture, so you should not get discouraged.

FIRST POSTURE: VRISHASANA (Bull posture)

EXECUTION: Sit down and bend the right leg under the left thigh. The right thigh should remain in the axis of the floor, the right leg should make a 45-degree angle with the left thigh. The left knee is upon the right one, as close as possible. The feet are symmetric from each side of the body. Place both hands upon the feet; the fingers are on each corresponding toe, the arms are straight and relaxed. Since the palms of the hands are on the soles of the feet, the circuit of energy is closed. Do a few complete breathing exercises and concentrate on the space between the two eyebrows (Ajna Chakra). After some time, release slowly the posture and reverse the position.

CONCENTRATION: Between the two eyebrows.

BREATHING: Complete and normal.

Before taking another posture by reversing the position of the legs, you can do in-between the next variant as described below.

SECOND POSTURE (variant):

This posture can be practiced right away after the first one before starting with another one.

EXECUTION: From the starting point sitting on the mat, the right leg remains folded under the left thigh, just as it is in the first posture. While taking a deep breath, lift up both arms vertically, hold the breath a few seconds, and then slowly bend your trunk towards your toes in exhaling, and try to catch them; the forehead should touch the left knee. Hold on the position with empty lungs as long as you can, and then bring up slowly the trunk while inhaling; Lift up again vertically both arms, exhale and bring them down. Reverse the posture and repeat it over again three or four times on each side.

CONCENTRATION: On the solar plexus, while holding the posture.

RESPIRATION RHYTHM: It should be deep and normal.

THERAPEUTIC RESULTS: The first posture is excellent for the nervous equilibrium and helps to develop concentration. A good tonic for the male sexual glands, it regularizes the circulation of the Pranic energy in the body.

SECOND POSTURE: It will extend and bring suppleness to the back muscles of the legs. A good tonic for the abdominal muscles will bring suppleness to the lumbar spine and may accelerate the healing of sciatica diseases.

VAJRASANA (Adamantine Posture)

This posture is similar to the adept one; the only differences is this: the student, instead of sitting on the ankles, is sitting between them, the buttocks on the floor. It is a little bit more difficult than the adept posture and cannot be accomplished until the adept one is mastered.

SAME CONCENTRATION AND SAME BREATHING

TRISTAMBHASANA (The sacred pillar posture)

This posture is not much comfortable for those with stiff legs. It also looks like the *Vajrasana*.

EXERCISE 1: Sitting on the heels, the knees are bent, but the toes instead of being flat on the floor, are bending. The bust is inclined backward, the arms straight with the hands touching the floor. The breathing is slow, and the concentration is on the thyroid gland.

EXERCISE 2: Sit on the heels just as in the previous posture, but this time keep the spine erect and the hands folded on the chest.

CONCENTRATION: On the heart (Anahat chakra)

Those two postures may cause in the beginning some discomforts in the toes, but soon, by practicing, it will disappear.

RESULTS: The first one has a tremendous effect on the thyroid gland by making it work better, and also on the joints of the knee, legs, and the toes. The second one is also beneficial for the joints of the knees, legs, toes, and it also helps for concentration.

PASCIMOTTANASANA (Posterior stretch posture)

This posture works very much on the back dorsal and on the legs, just like the one described in the previous lesson. In this one only the position of the hands is changed. Instead of catching the ankles, catch each big toe of the feet with the index of each hand, and try to make the forehead touch the knees without bending them. This posture is a little bit more difficult than the one described before, and should be performed only when the previous one is mastered.

RESULTS: Same breathing, same concentration, and same therapeutic values.

Note: For more understanding, you should refer yourself to the stretch posture described in the second part of the second lesson.

BHUNAMANAVAJRASANA (Worship posture)

This exercise is between Asana (posture) and Mudra (symbolic gestures.)

EXECUTION: It is performed from the *Vajrasana*, or the adamantine posture. Kneel down and sit on the heel with the bust erect and try to catch the wrist of one hand with the other hand placed behind the back. Take a deep breath, and then bend your bust forward slowly while exhaling, and keep on going down until your forehead touches the floor.

DETAILED EXPLANATIONS: Stay in the posture with empty lungs, and then come up slowly while inhaling. Exhale when the bust is vertical. You can also remain in the posture while breathing slowly but ceding three minutes.

CONCENTRATION: On the Anahat chakra.

VARIANT: You can also separate the legs and the knees. For that, bend yourself forward, but the buttocks should not leave the heel. This posture requires a little bit more suppleness of the ankles than the previous one.

RESULTS: It brings suppleness to the lumbar region, will bring relief to sciatica diseases, acts upon the organs of the abdominal cavity, and assure a powerful positive mental effect.

BHUJANGASANA (Cobra posture)

This is a basic posture which should be practiced every day. In *Halasana* (the plough posture), described in the fourth lesson, the back muscles are stretched to the maximum, while the front muscles are contracted. In the *Bhujangasana* (cobra posture), the contrary is done; the front muscles are stretched to the maximum. Both postures are complementary.

EXECUTION: Lying down on your belly, keep both feet together with the hands flat on the floor near the shoulders. First, empty the lungs by exhaling, and then while inhaling lift up your head and bend the bust backward with the help of your back muscles.

From the head to the lumbar region, the spine is curved. Stretch farther the movement with the help of your hands, until the navel region lifts off the floor. Keep the posture for approximately six to twelve seconds, while holding the breath, and then slowly come back to the starting position in exhaling. Repeat the posture three to six times.

In the beginning, if the respiratory rhythm does not suit you, hold your breath for a couple of seconds or breathe normally. In this way, you will be able to keep the posture for a longer period of time.

THERAPEUTIC EFFECTS: It brings suppleness to the front muscles and strength to the back ones, and may correct the defect of the back and spine. It also helps in the better function of the thyroid gland.

MENTAL CONCENTRATION: Upon the thyroid gland. The concentration could also be on the nerves of spinal column.

RESPIRATION RHYTHM: It is already described with the exercise. However, you can just observe the breathing if you retain the breath. If you do not, keep a slow and normal breathing.

వ

LESSON 3 PART 2
THE SCIENCE OF PRANAYAMA

RHYTHMICAL PRANAYAMA WITH RETENTION

Do not forget the careful advice about pranayama that we have already given you in the second part of the second lesson. Please read it again.

EXECUTION: Sit down in any comfortable posture, after exhaling to empty the lungs, take a complete inhalation without forcing, but instead of exhaling right away, hold on the breath and focus the concentration on the heart or Anahat chakra. After the retention, let the air go out slowly through both nostrils.

THE LENGTH OF TIME IN THIS EXERCISE: You should start during the first week with a rhythm of 3-6-6. Those numbers are for the timing of the seconds. The first one is for the inhalation, which should be done for 3 seconds. The next one is for the retention (6 seconds), and the third number is for the expiration. This exercise should be repeated 3 to 4 times.

As you are progressing and as your respiratory system is getting used to it, you should increase the rhythm to 4-8-8, then 5-10-10, and then up to 6-12-12, after three weeks of practice.

After about one month of regular practice, if you are feeling comfortable while doing this pranayama, you can modify the rhythm by adopting a new one in which the length of time of the retention is four times longer than the inhalation.

Starting from 3-12-6 seconds, and after some time, you will decide yourself to go further with 4-16-8, and then 6-24-12 to reach 8-32-16, which should be the maximum for most ordinary students. Those who are suffering from any slight heart condition and blood pressure problems should not exceed 3-12-6 seconds.

Those who are suffering from other minor respiratory problems should practice this pranayama with discretion and according to their own possibilities. Anyway, if you are feeling any discomfort or pain in the chest region, instead of increasing the length of time, on the contrary you should decrease it or stop the practice. Any respiratory exercises should start after completely emptying the lungs.

CONCENTRATION: It should be focused on the time length of the rhythm, while the prana is directed in different parts of the body according to its needs (heart, kidneys).

RETENTION WITH EMPTY LUNGS

Sit down in any comfortable posture or *Sukhasana* after completely emptying the lungs. Immediately take a deep inhalation and follow with a total exhalation. Before inhaling again, with empty lungs hold the breath for approximately 6 to 12 seconds. But in fact, after a complete inhalation, the yogis believe that a remainder of about 1.5 liters of air is still in the lungs, which is sufficient to keep up the oxygenation of the blood. If you feel any discomfort in the chest region, reduce right away the length of time of the retention.

CONCENTRATION: On the whole health of the body.

After some time of pranayama practices with breath retention, the results soon are felt. Just as in the previous breathing exercise we have described, the blood circulation is improving, and the cells are getting more oxygenation from the blood. The heart is relaxing, the skin complexion is getting brighter, the eyes are clearer, and the tone of the voice is getting warmer and more sonorous. The nervous system is more relaxed, and the entire metabolism is improving.

PSYCHIC RESULTS: The memory is improving, the Spirit is getting sharper, and intuition is developing. Mental concentration is becoming easier, and the spiritual faculties are awakening. However, keep in mind that all of those claimed achievements will not happen to you within a few days or months. You have to keep practicing honestly and regularly for a long time.

ℒ

LESSON 3   **PART 3**

HIGHER YOGA
The Way to the Discovery

The higher yoga is for those who have decided to regularize their lives with the help of the yoga discipline. Through this discipline the physical and emotional body will slowly be purified by obtaining mastery over them. They no longer will constitute as obstacles to the discovery of the higher self.

However, after mastering the psychological emotional aspect of the physical body, another obstacle will remain, which is the *mental barrier*, the most powerful one surrounding the Spirit. The kingdom of light, truth, and beatitude is beyond the lower mental agitation. The mastery over the mind will be the most difficult task for one to achieve. It might take you several months or many births to master the mind. However, it depends on one's own degree of spiritual evolution of karma. You cannot expect any real spiritual contact until you are able to control the various thought waves entering the mind. Usually in higher yoga, the yogi needs to surrender to his or her own inner self in order to achieve that goal.

We insist on the difficulty you will experience to control and eventually to master the mind. You should not get discouraged. Just as in hatha yoga, you should arm yourself with the three great virtues: patience, perseverance, and willpower.

CONCENTRATION: The first step toward meditation

In the first part of the second lesson, you have studied concentration. It is very important in the practice of hatha yoga. We already have explained that it also leads to the step of higher yoga. It is this step that we are now about to approach.

Let us take the mental concentration as it has been described in the second lesson, which you should review. We have said that you need to first stop the constant flow of your thoughts, and then with the help of the willpower, focus the attention on one point and try to keep it there.

FIRST – CONCENTRATION ON ONE OBJECT

This is one of the simplest forms of concentration. For example, take a flower and try to scrutinize it thoroughly. All your thoughts should be directed only towards it. Look at its form, its colors, appreciate its weight, its smell; notice all the details of its constitution, such as the stalk, the sepals, the petals, the stamens, and the pistil. Feel the delicacy of the petals, and count them up. During all these observations, your thoughts and your concentration will be converted only upon the flower. No other thoughts should occupy the mind. You can enhance the concentration by focusing the mind upon one element of the flower, which you will study (the pistil, for example). You will then reduce the field of your consciousness to one point. After that, you can choose another object and concentrate upon it according to the same techniques. You can also multiply the number of the objects as much as you want.

You can also choose a geometrical figure or a symbol as the focus of the concentration. For example, make use of a triangle, a square, a circle, a spiral, a lotus form, a pentagram, or the cross.

SECOND – VISUALIZATION

In another step, after you have trained yourself to concentrate upon one object, you will close your eyes and then try to recreate mentally your object in all of its details, without having it near you. By doing this, you will enter into a very important field of the mind—the form creation, which is included in higher steps of superior initiations.

You will train yourself to observe different objects and to reproduce their images in your mind with closed eyes. You can also try to recreate through the memory a painting or a landscape which you have seen in the past.

THIRD – MENTAL CONCENTRATION ON ONE IDEA

We are taking you into a new step of concentration. In this one, instead of focusing on one object, do it upon an idea. You will notice that it is more difficult to concentrate upon an abstract idea than to concentrate on one concrete object apprehensible by the senses. The idea belongs to the mental field—it does not have any sensory basis—and this is its main difficulty.

However, you should persevere and train yourself regularly. Choose as the subject of your concentration these virtues: Goodness, Universal Love, Truth, Purity, Spiritual Determination. Such concentration has the advantage to elevate your feelings and to direct your entire being towards the virtues you have chosen and to make you further notable progress. You can also concentrate your thoughts upon the spiritual light you hope to discover. In that way, you will prepare the mind for the more difficult higher stages of meditation.

FOURTH – EMPTINESS OF THE MIND

One more step into the mind field is to empty it from all thoughts. This also is a little difficult to achieve, but not impossible, and is a must in order to develop contemplation. To succeed, you have to chase out the thoughts before they invade deeply the mind. In fact, one can empty the mind only for a few seconds, only very advanced yogis in Samadhi are able to empty the mind for a long time. Just as nature, which cannot remain empty, the ordinary mind, as soon as thoughts are eliminated, gives automatically birth to new ones.

The goal in achieving higher thoughts is to order the thoughts in such a manner that the lower negative thoughts (*Rajasic* or *Tamasic*) are constantly eliminated and replaced by positive, elevating (*Satwic*) thoughts in order to permit the descent of superior mental manifestation in the consciousness.

During the practice, the first exercises are usually disappointing, but one should not get discouraged. Many have declared that it is impossible to empty the mind, because they did not have enough patience to further their efforts. In the beginning, ridiculous thoughts will come to replace those you have chased out. If you persevere in your efforts, the thoughts which will come to fill the empty mind will be more and more of a higher grade. You will have to feel the descent of the spiritual light and the subtle energies. When that stage is reached, know then that you are nearer to contemplation. Remember this great word of the Master: "Empty thyself completely, and I shall fill thee up."

Exercise yourself in a calm place away from any kind of disturbances. Sit comfortably with a light stomach, preferably during the same hours, and relax yourself. This step that prepares for mental concentration may take time to master, but you should not get discouraged. In the next lesson, we will try to initiate you into meditation.

Meditation is the basis of spiritual activities, which should be part of your life style. It could become really useful to you, when you will be able to master concentration. You should then exercise the mind to those two activities until the concentration stage is over and to stabilize definitely the mind into the practice of meditation.

CHAPTER VI

THE MORAL CODE IN YOGA (YAMA – NIYAMA)

Yoga, as it has been practiced in India for thousands of years has a moral code, a life discipline which proves that it has a spiritual end. Moral rules and a proper life discipline are necessary for complete success in yoga. We have already explained those problems in the third part of our second lesson. Please review again the above-mentioned lesson. Those who wish to practice the higher yoga must follow absolutely the moral code of yoga. Those who are practicing yoga only for health and physical fitness do not necessarily have to follow all the moral rules of yoga. However, we must point out to you what it is all about, in order that those who wish to follow them can do so and be fully aware of their advantages.

We have to remind you that exoteric hatha yoga can be practiced with good results without observing the moral code, but their observances can only enhance the success of the result. Lastly, it is up to each individual practitioner to decide their best option. By the way, some asanas and pranayama's cannot be safely practiced without observing the moral rules and a proper diet.

The first of the rules is: **NON-VIOLENCE** - A yoga sadhaka should not annoy anyone in thoughts, speech, and action

TRUTHFULNESS IN SPEECH – The sadhaka should avoid telling lies at any cost and truth must be his or her law. One should live a simple life, self-contented with no desire for others' properties. One should maintain internal and external purity and cleanliness of the body.

One must try to reach a stage of mental impartiality, and learn to understand the right view of the events of life. Most of the things in the world which attract our attention have little value in the eternal play. The yogi must learn to see the events of life just as they are coming and going in reality, but not as they are interpreted by the ordinary human mind. The yogi should not be affected by them, as most of the people are.

One should reach the stage of non-reaction to the trouble of life. One should struggle to always keep a balanced mind in all circumstances. The yogi's speech, actions, and whatever is taking place must be under control.

The sadhaka must always focus on self-studies and the study of the scripture in order to know the self better.

The sadhaka must surrender to the divine power of God, according to his or her own ideas.

Now remember, those moral rules are written in the yoga scriptures, and they are only for the serious yoga seekers who are contemplating to achieving higher goals in the holistic yoga knowledge. Those of you who are only expecting physical suppleness and some ability to concentrate should not necessarily pay attention to the rules, mostly if you feel that those rules could not fit into your life style.

∽

LESSON 4   PART 2
THE ASANAS (Postures)

This lesson is particularly important; please study it carefully. You will study during the next fifteen days three main asanas: *Swastika Asana* (Swastika Posture), *Halasanasana* (Plough Posture) and *Dhanushasana* (Bow Posture)

These asanas are among those you should keep practicing regularly and every day. We will also study alternate breathing, which is one of the most effective pranayama. However, you should continue to perfect the exercises in the previous lessons, which should have their place in your daily yoga session. The triangular postures which are in this lesson are also very important. Here are twelve advices, some of which have already been given. Read them carefully and always keep them in mind whenever you are practicing yoga.

TWELVE ADVICES TO THE SADHAKA

1. Yoga must be practiced on hard ground. You should use a folded blanket, a yoga mat, or a carpet. Never practice on a bed/water bed.

2. Yoga is a psycho-physical self-discipline. It requires a silent atmosphere, calmness, relaxation of the body and the spirit.

3. Haste is the enemy of yoga. Slowness is the key. Yoga is the contrary of Western gymnastic or regular DVD or TV workout programs.

4. Patience, perseverance, and willpower are necessary. Without them you may not succeed in becoming a yogi. It takes at least three to six months to start feeling the beneficial effects of yoga.

5. A yoga session should be practiced at least two hours after food. Intestines and bladders should not be overloaded. The sitting postures can be practiced at any time.

6. You should not feel tired after a yoga session; on the contrary, the body should feel relaxed with plenty of energy. If it is not so, that means you are not practicing properly.

7. Mostly after practicing a series of stretching asanas, you should always relax in *Shavasana*.

8. While performing the asanas, correct breathing and concentration must be carefully observed.

9. In the beginning, the difficult postures should be practiced daily, but one should never force the limbs. After some time, notable progress will automatically come.

10. Some difficult postures must be practiced with great care in order not to hurt oneself. If you keep this in mind along with the rule of slowness, you will avoid many troubles.

11. You should also be careful with the practice of pranayama, mostly with kumbaka, or breath retention. You should progressively count the length of time of the exercises.

12. After each session of pranayama, you should remain in the sitting position for at least five minutes in order to absorb the prana thoroughly in the body.

THE ANGLE POSTURE (Konasana)
FIRST POSTURE:

EXECUTION: Standing up, separate the legs from each other at about two and a half feet. Bring up the arms in a lateral position until they reach the horizontal with the palms of the hands turning upward.

Take a deep breath, and then slowly bend the trunk downward, the right hand touches the left foot if possible. Turn your neck to the left and look at your left hand raising up. Keep the posture while holding your breath with empty lungs as long as you can. You come up slowly to the horizontal position, while inhaling, and then bring the arms downward near the body in exhaling. Wait a few seconds before starting the same exercise on the opposite side.

CONCENTRATION: On the spinal column at the lumbar region.

RESPIRATORY RHYTHM: Brings suppleness to the lateral muscles of the trunk, the back, and the hips. Enhances the intestine peristaltic and prevents constipation. It also massages the liver and strengthens the lumbar spine.

SECOND POSTURE (Variant)

In this variant, take the same position with the same breathing, but the right hand will touch the right foot instead of the opposite one, and the left hand will rise up. Afterwards, reverse the position. Repeat three to six times each side. This exercise is giving a great workout to the hips, and therefore may considerably help in melting out fat.

SWASTIKASANA (Swastika Posture)

This posture of great stability cannot be easily done until the *Sukhasana* is mastered. Up to now, if you are not able to perform it correctly, you should continue with the previous suppleness posture before doing the Swastika. In this case you should adopt *Vajrasana* (the adamantine posture), or the tailor one, which will help you better to keep the spinal column well erect in order to practice pranayama and meditation.

EXECUTION: Sit down just as in *Sukhasana*, bend the right leg, the ball and the heel of the right foot against the left thigh. Keep the heel near the perineum. Bend the left leg, then catch the left foot with the right hand, and place it upon the calf of the right leg. The toes of the right foot should come out between the thigh and the left leg to better stabilize the posture. Keep the spinal column in the vertical position and the hands are relaxing on the knees. After some time reverse the position of the legs.

CONCENTRATION: On the leg muscles and upon the heart region.

RESULTS: After constant practice, this posture will become a relaxed sitting one. It is used for the practice of meditation and pranayama. It is also an excellent tonic for mental equilibrium.

HALASANA (Plough Posture)

This is also a basic posture which should be practiced carefully and regularly.

PRELIMINARY ADVICES: *Halasana* should be practiced very carefully. After a certain age, the spinal column has lost its full suppleness; therefore, you must proceed cautiously with slow movement and stop at once whenever you start feeling some uncomfortable pain. In the beginning, you may feel some apprehension; you then should help yourself with some pillows or a small chair by placing the feet upon them, and which should be taken away as soon as the feet are touching the floor. You should avoid jerking and discontinue as soon as the tension becomes too much on the neck and shoulder muscles. It might happen in the first performances that the feet cannot touch the floor, but you should not give up and think that it is impossible to do. You should be confident that one day the spinal column will get enough suppleness to assure you the posture.

EXECUTION: Lie down on the back, the arms alongside the body, and keep the hands flat on the floor. Lift up both legs slowly into the vertical position, and then bend them toward your head. Keep both feet close to each other. The pelvis and the trunk should follow the movement. You should try to touch the floor with the toes. The arms and the hands remain flat on the floor. In the beginning, you may feel some tension around the neck, and then you should not stay too long in the position. Watch your head, which should remain exactly in the axis of the body. By doing this, you will avoid a sprain in the neck. While performing the exercise, you may feel less breathing and a little bit uncomfortable in the throat region. You should then breathe slowly and regularly through the abdominal.

When you are able to touch the floor with the toes, you should straighten the legs as much as you can in order to increase the flexion of the spinal column. Do not bend the knees. Keep the posture as long as you can without any discomfort. Afterward, come back into the initial position by some reverse and slow movements. You should never come up right away after doing the posture. On the contrary, you need to take rest in *Shavasana*.

If you want to do the *Halasana* from the oblique posture, or *Ardha-Halasana*, you just have to keep the arms and the hands flat on the floor. Take the support of them in order to bring the legs slowly toward your head, until the toes touch the floor. You must be careful while performing the asanas, as we have previously advised you.

BREATHING: Normally through the abdomen.

CONCENTRATION: Upon the spinal column.

THERAPEUTIC RESULTS: This posture is one of the best yoga postures. It may correct the deviations of the spinal column. It appears that it reacts upon the entire endocrine system: the pituitary gland, the thyroid, the pancreas, the thymus, the genital glands, and the adrenal glands. It vivifies the entire glandular system.

VISTRITA-PADA SARVANGASANA (Spread-Out Feet And Limbs)
After you have mastered *Halasana* you can, from the *Sarvangasana* position, increase the flexion of the spinal column by spreading out the legs as much as you can without losing your balance. This posture is more difficult than the previous one and should not be attempted until *Halasana* can be performed with ease.

SAME BREATHING, SAME CONCENTRATION, SAME THERAPEUTIC EFFECTS.

GOMUKHASANA (Cow Head Posture)
EXECUTION: Sit between the legs spread out and the knees on the floor. Bend one arm on the back. Pass the other arm above the shoulder and try to catch the hands.

CONCENTRATION: On the posture

BREATHING: Normal and regular.

RESULTS: This exercise gives suppleness to the joints of the shoulders, strengthens the trapezius muscles, and develops the rib cage. For those with short arms, it might be quite uneasy to perform, but with regular practice you might be able to overcome this disadvantage.

SETUVASANA (Bridge Posture)

EXECUTION: Lie down, keeping the hands alongside the body. Bend the knees a little bit with the feet close to each other and flat on the floor. First, take the support of the feet, the shoulders, and then the head. Bring the body up while bending the spinal column as much as you can. Place the hands under the hips and the elbows on the floor to help maintain the posture. Breathe normally and keep the position as long as you can, and then take rest in *Shavasana.*

CONCENTRATION: On the spinal column

THERAPEUTIC RESULTS: It brings suppleness to the spinal column in extension, and strengthens the muscles of the trunk and the neck. Excellent for women with pelvic problems

RESPIRATION: While holding the posture, it should be slow and regular.

PREPARATION FOR MATSYENDRASANA

In order to perform easily *Matsyendrasana*, it is better to proceed step by step.

Let us study the first step of this posture. For those students who still have a stout body, they may first adopt the posture we are about to describe if later on they are unable to master the *Matsyendrasana.*

EXECUTION: Take a sitting position; bend the left leg, keep the left thigh in the axis of the floor, and the left heel is against the right buttock. Bring the right leg upon the left thigh; keep the right foot flat on the floor against the left knee. The right leg is vertical, and the right thigh is pressing the abdomen. Keep the arms relaxed on each side of the body with the hands on the floor with straight fingers, the arms making a 45-degree angle with the body. Try to stay motionless in this posture, breathe slowly and completely. After some time, slowly reverse the position of the legs.

MENTAL CONCENTRATION: On the heart center.

THERAPEUTIC RESULTS: This posture is proven to be good for physical and mental balance. It also brings suppleness to the hips and may correct the defects of the spinal column.

THE GREAT PRAYER POSTURE (Variant of Bhunamanavajrasana)

EXECUTION: Sit in the adept posture (on the heels, the knees on the ground), lift up your arms vertically while inhaling. Bend the body slowly forward with the arms as they are and exhale until the hands touch the floor. Keep the position a few seconds with empty lungs. While holding the posture, keep on stretching the hands on the floor in order to make the articulations of the shoulder work more. After some time, come up while inhaling, with straight arms. Exhale and bring the arms down alongside the body. Repeat the posture three times.

CONCENTRATION: On the movement of the exercise.

BREATHING: Observe carefully the respiratory rhythm which has been indicated in the posture.

THERAPEUTIC RESULTS: It gives suppleness to the lumbar region. It is also an ideal posture to correct sciatica. In addition, it brings suppleness to the back and the shoulder muscles. It may also produce a positive psychic effect.

DHANUSHASANA (Bow Posture)

This is the third basic posture of the fourth lesson.

EXECUTION: Lying on the belly, bend both knees, and try to catch the ankles. While inhaling, bend your torso, keep the arms straight, raise the head and the trunk, and hold the breath. The knees have left the ground. Hold the posture for a few second, and then come back in the initial position while exhaling and still holding the legs. After a few seconds of rest, start over the posture. After each period of rest, you may repeat it three to four times.

CONCENTRATION: Upon the lumbar region.

BREATHING: As prescribed in the exercise.

THERAPEUTIC RESULTS: Supposedly, it should produce a powerful beneficial effect upon the endocrine glands. It is also beneficial to the liver and the spleen. It has a powerful effect on the nervous centers of the spinal column. The stretching effect of this exercise may also reduce the effect of cellulitis of the abdomen, the hips, and the legs.

THE SCIENCE OF BREATHING (Pranayama)
THE ALTERNATE PRANAYAMA, OR ANULUM VILUM

We are going to study this type of pranayama, which is shown to produce some positive effect upon the nervous system.

The practice of the alternate pranayama cleans the passage of both nostrils, stabilizes the current of energy in the body, and reduces agitation.

EXECUTION: Sit in any comfortable posture. First empty the lungs by exhaling from both nostrils. Close the right nostril with the thumb of the right hand. Inhale deeply and slowly through the left nostril. Close the left nostril with the index and the major finger of the right-hand, and then exhale completely through the right nostril. Without moving the two fingers, inhale through the right nostril. Close again the right nostril with the thumb, and liberate the left one in which you exhale. Once more, inhale through the left nostril and exhale through both.

This complete cycle is count for one pranayama. You should repeat it 4 to 6 times and then take rest, while breathing normally.

THERAPEUTIC EFFECTS: It stabilizes the positive and the negative currents in the body. It helps clean the lungs, calm down the nervous system. It also helps in preparing the mind for concentration and meditation.

CONCENTRATION: While performing the exercise, concentrate upon the coming and going of the air in the nostril. Imagine the purified air which is spreading all over the cells of the brain. In order to become more proficient in pranayama, you need to continue with the practice of complete breathing, and master the Kumbakha Pranayama we have already taught. Practice regularly this new pranayama, which is very important, and increase the length of time as you are progressing and feeling more comfortable.

అ

LESSON 4   **PART 3**

HIGHER YOGA

We are now going to study one of the most important steps in higher yoga: meditation and concentration.

Meditation is the highest spiritual activity of a sadhaka, which should be practiced continuously in order to maintain contact with the cosmic consciousness. In the same way, the body lives with air; in breathing, the spirit lives with meditation. Meditation is a vital activity of the superior vehicles within us. By the practice of it, one raises oneself above the material plane and reaches the high Spirit. Meditation helps to create a channel of light in which the subtle energies come down and flow into the lower vehicles, progressively achieving their mutation. All of the great beings who have lived on this planet have considered meditation as their daily food.

MEDITATION

The success of this activity depends on certain basic physical conditions.

THE PHYSICAL CONDITIONS:

THE PLACE: You need to choose a quiet room where you will not be disturbed. It is better to try to meditate in the same room in order to get it saturated with your own vibrations. The yogi considers the meditation room as a holy place where only higher thoughts are entertained. One should not eat or smoke in that room. This room is not a meeting place, and anyone with no spiritual purpose should not be allowed to enter that room. In order to maintain the positive vibration, you may want to keep in it the images of great masters or saints of your choice, and to burn incense.

THE MOMENT: You should train yourself to meditate always at the same time in order to develop a favorable automation. The best moments are early in the morning after getting up, and at night before or two hours after food. However, each person may have different preferences; therefore, plan your meditation sessions according to your own lifestyle and choose an hour which suits you the best. Note: according to certain yogic traditions, special moments particularly favorable for meditation coincide with different phases of the moon: the day of the full moon, and the day of the new moon. The preceding day and the day which follow those two moments of the lunar cycle are very special for meditation.

THE PHYSIOLOGICAL CONDITION: The body needs to be healthy, relaxed, and calm. Meditation should be practiced at a certain distance between meals, which should be light. Physical discomfort with muscular tension should be first subdued with a session of hatha yoga. In a good meditation, a sadhaka should feel relaxed, and forget about the existence of the body. For those with agitated mind, it is recommended to start meditation by listening to soft, relaxed music.

THE POSTURE: Long experience has proven that a good posture for meditation is the one which helps maintain the spinal column in the vertical position in order for the magnetic current drawn in meditation to circulate freely. In addition, the spinal column must be free from tension. It is for this reason that the yogis considered that the most suitable yoga postures for meditation are the following: *Siddhasana, Sukhasana,* and *Padmasana*. However, a student who is unable to sit comfortably in any of those positions may use an arm chair with a straight back. While sitting on a chair, keep the spine erect, the head straight, with closed eyes, with the hands relaxed on the knees or folded. One should remain completely relaxed; however, in the beginning it is advised not to meditate in *Shavasana* or lying down, which may lead you to sleep.

THE BREATHING: The respiratory rhythm is very important in bringing to the mind the state of relaxation and peace. It should be in harmony with the current of thoughts. The breathing which should be adopted for meditation is the complete slow breathing we have described in the first lesson.

THE PRACTICAL TECHNIQUE OF MEDITATION

MEDITATION UPON AN IDEA: Without concentration, no real meditation is possible. It is for this reason that you must train yourself daily and for a long time to the practice of concentration, as it has been taught previously. From the stage of concentration which does not allow any foreign thoughts to intervene in the chosen subject, you should start with the process of meditation by studying the subject in all of its aspects.

In other words, you are analyzing the subject. You are doing a kind of mental dissection. The great ideas upon which you already have learnt to concentrate in the previous lesson could be some kind of themes for your meditation. If you try to understand them, you will develop higher thoughts. Those ideas are part of the cosmic consciousness. By adjusting them with your mental and spiritual way of living, you will arrive closer to the cosmic consciousness. Those ideas could serve as a bridge between the matter and the Spirit. Truth, universal love, and wisdom are the great subjects upon which one can orient the meditation in the beginning.

A SUPERIOR STAGE OF MEDITATION

From the emptiness of the mind comes a higher state of meditation. It is that superior state of meditation which one day you should try to achieve. It is possible to inspire you with some rules and techniques to reach that goal. According to each sadhaka, the method may be different. We will try to give you a few hints in the hope that they will help you as they have helped us. You need to understand that we are entering a realm where the language can only explain partially the reality. It is difficult to communicate the experiences of meditation through the experiences of the material world, as they are not suitable for explaining the experiences of the spiritual world.

THE REFERENCE POINTS:

The silence of three inferior vehicles—physical, emotional, and mental—is indispensable. If one of them gets excited, soon you will be back on the material plan.

An effort is necessary to establish the contact, a vertical effort, an effusion.

The effusion must be at the same time an opening to the cosmic forces or the above spiritual forces.

The consciousness must remain open and alert for the descent of higher forces, but mental thoughts must be stable.

If you have decided to go toward the cosmic consciousness, it will come to you. In fact, the cosmic consciousness is eternally present; it is the human who does not make the effort to discover it.

You may also ask this question to yourself: who am I? Then you should try to get rid of the obstacle of lower mental thoughts, until the intuitive answer comes from the higher superior plane.

You can concentrate on a light point at the center of the head. It is from there that illumination and the descent of higher energies will come. Light will attract light.

Study carefully each of those different points, and try to understand how they can be adjusted to your particular case.

We have to remind you that meditation must be a lifetime activity for you. Even the great beings who attained the highest peak of spiritual fulfillment continue to meditate.

THE CONTEMPLATION

Contemplation is the highest step. One must have practiced meditation in many previous births in order to reach that stage of unification with cosmic consciousness. During meditation, the forces which came down have the power to transform the lower vehicles and to increase the vibratory rhythm. When the personal consciousness has disappeared or melted itself into the cosmic consciousness, the goal is achieved. It is that stage which Western mystics called "Ecstasy," and in yoga, it is known as "Samadhi" or "Ecstasy." It is known that very few can reach that stage. Those who are blessed by such transcendental experience have access to all knowledge. They come back to the physical plane enlightened.

We cannot give any advice, nor can any technique be taught or described, to achieve that stage. Contemplation is the reward of many births of pure life dedicated to love, meditation, and higher Spirit.

If one does not have the ambition to reach the supreme goal because it seems too difficult, one should not forget that meditation is already a high step which can satisfy all desires in life. It will prepare the entire being for further realizations.

CHAPTER VII

PRELIMINARY NOTIONS ON MUSCLES
AND ARTICULATIONS

T HE MUSCLES – Schematically, the muscles are masses of flesh which are attached to the bones by their tendons, and in this way permit the movement of the body (movement of different limbs, the neck, and the trunk).

In this chapter, we are giving only a brief description of the skeletal muscles and how they are affected by hatha yoga exercises, according to Indian yoga masters. One of the essential characteristics of the muscles is to be resilient. The property is enhanced by the practice of the yoga postures. The goal of the asanas is to maintain or restore the elasticity of the muscular fibers in the body.

The muscles are excitable and contractible by nervous influx. This last property of the muscles permits them to move the bony levers and to assure the movements and the attitudes of the body. By doing any physical activity, the muscles are using energy. This energy is generated by food, particularly the carbohydrate. The contraction of the muscles generates heat and energy. The wastes which are produced by important hard work, in the form of lactic acid, may bring stiffness to the body (Roth, S.M. 2006).

THE VARIOUS MUSCLES WHICH MAY BE AFFECTED
BY YOGA ASANAS

According to the yogic literature, the yoga asanas make mostly all of the muscles work.

THE PRINCIPAL MUSCLES OF THE ANTERIOR PART
OF THE TRUNK.

THE BIG PECTORAL MUSCLES – It covers the chest, and the end of its tendon is attached upon the humerus, or the arm bone.

THE ABDOMEN MUSCLES – There are four which are upon each other. From the deep plane, they are successively:

1. Transversal Abdominal 2. Internal oblique 3. External oblique 4. Pectoralis Major.

All those muscles are affected by a great number of asanas, either in contraction or elongation. The transverse muscles are raised up.

2. THE PRINCIPAL MUSCLES ON THE POSTERIOR PLANE:

The spinal muscles, which are attached to the spinal column. The main ones are the sacro-lumbar mass and the long dorsal, which goes up to the cervical vertebra.

The great dorsal muscle which is spread in the back with the final tendons attached upon the humerus.

The trapezius muscle, which covers the scapular and the neck.

All those muscles quoted are affected by many asanas, mostly of those which make the spinal cord bend or extend. These postures will prolong and make supple the muscular masses and the tendons upon which the muscles are attached on the bone.

3.THE SUPERIOR MUSCLES OF THE LIMBS:

The Deltoid, which has three bundles upon the shoulder and makes the arms move.

The Biceps, which bends the forearm upon the arm.

The Triceps, which spreads the forearm when it is bent by the biceps.

4.THE INFERIOR MUSCLES OF THE LIMBS:

The Psoas-Iliac, or hip bone muscles, which bend the thigh.

The Big Buttock, which spreads the thigh (Those two muscles are together attached on the femur and the iliac bone).

The Three Muscles Ischium-Tibia, which make the leg bend on the thigh.

The Quadriceps Muscle, made of four muscles, which make the leg spread when it is bent.

Those different muscles are affected by the sitting postures, as well as the feet and leg muscles.

The Posterior Leg Muscles, which lift up the feet.

The Triceps Sural Muscle, which stretches the feet.

Indeed, the yoga asanas are beneficial even if you ignore the name, the place, and the purpose of the muscle involved. However, for the serious student who wants to practice safely the science of yoga, it is recommended to know where the muscles involved in the posture are located in the body, and how they are functioning in this complex human machine. In this manner, you can follow with accuracy the work of the muscles for better results of the asanas.

Finally, let us remind you of the key muscle in the respiratory system, THE DIAPHRAGM, which we already have studied in a previous lesson.

THE ARTICULATIONS

The articulations are the way to unite the bones. They allow the movements of different bony segments by the media of the muscles. We distinguish between the motionless articulations, semi-mobile, and mobile. In yoga, we are interested only in mobile articulations. In this chapter, we leave aside the very important articulations of the spinal cord. We shall deal with them in a special chapter.

In dealing with the complexity of the human body, the spinal column is considered as the support of the whole body, which preoccupies mostly the science of yoga. Added to it are other connecting articulations which are much involved in the postures, such as the hips, the knees, the ankles, the shoulders, the elbows, and the wrists.

Those six articulations have a common characteristic in their structures. It is important for a sadhaka to know even in a summary way how an articulation is formed, in order to understand how they are affected by the postures and in order to maintain their elasticity and their good physiological functioning.

ARTICULATION DESCRIPTION

The end of the bones, which are the constituent of the articulations, are covered with cartilage, a firm elastic tissue which permits the sliding of the two articulate surfaces of one against the other.

The articular capsule is a fibrous membrane which unites the bones. It is attached at the periphery of the cartilage. It is covered with a tissue secreting a lubricious liquid called synovial fluid which helps to diagnose the cause of joint inflammation (Morrison, W.A. 2015).

The ligaments are some thin fiber blades binding the bones together to prevent them from splitting. They are attached to the bones and sometimes come to the capsule. The yoga postures act upon the ligaments to stretch them and to maintain their suppleness. They also react upon the articular capsule in the same way to delay the aging process. In this process, the blood is circulating properly, and the cartilages remain alive. By the practice of yoga, the symptoms of rheumatism are controlled, and regular yoga practice may even delay its appearance.

❧

LESSON 5   **PART 2**

THE POSTURES, OR ASANAS

In this lesson, we will introduce two new basic postures, after which you will have all the necessary elements to practice a complete yoga session. In the last two months, you have begun the practice of yoga with us. As you figure out the cumulative balance, you will notice that after this fifth lesson you have learned twelve basic essential postures, which you need to practice daily. We feel that those basic postures could make up the entire physical yoga necessary for the average yoga seekers. They are sufficient to maintain the elasticity of the spinal cord, the articulations, the muscles, and to invigorate the endocrine system, and to maintain general good health.

However, it is also recommended to add the pranayama's you have learned, which are very important, along with mental concentration. We do not mean that the other asanas and pranayamas are useless. They are less important for ordinary students. But it is in your interest to know and to practice from time to time all the other asanas and pranayamas of hatha yoga, which will be taught in the next lessons. Please keep in mind that all the yoga postures and pranayamas in the holistic yoga have their importance in the human complex.

We understand that all yoga aspirants do not have the same goal. With the modern way of living, one may not be in a position to devote much time to the yoga practice. You should make a choice. Practice daily the basic postures, and add to your sessions one or two postures of the next lesson, which will be taught, and it is the same for pranayama.

THE TRIANGULAR POSTURES (Konasana And Variants)

FIRST POSTURE: N.B. – See the description of the simple triangular posture in the previous lesson (Lesson 4 Part 2).

EXECUTION: Just like the simple triangular posture.

DIFFERENCE: On the side where the body is inclined, the leg should be bent; the arm behind the knee and the hand is resting on the floor.

BREATHING: Same as in the simple triangular posture.

CONCENTRATION: Also the same

SECOND POSTURE (Variant)

Just as in the simple triangular posture, the body is twisted. First bend the leg on the other side, pass the arm in the front of the bent knee, and let the hand rest on the floor; the other arm is in a vertical position.

BREATHING: The same, concentration as well.

RESULTS: Same as in the simple posture, but somewhat more effective (see Lesson 4, Part 2).

THE BENT TREE POSTURE (Vakrikrita-Vrikshasana)

See again the description of the posture in Lesson 3, Part 2. This posture is performed from the second variant of the tree posture.

EXECUTION: In the tree posture, the foot is turned, and the heel is placed upon the thigh near the joint, the arms raised up vertically. Bend forward the arms and the bust, without losing your balance. You should reach the floor with straight fingers or the hands flat on the floor. Keep the position as long as you can and come back up slowly. After some rest, start again the posture and reverse the legs. Repeat the exercise three to four times on each side.

BREATHING: Inhale while lifting up the arms. Exhale while bending forward to the floor. Hold the breath with empty lungs, then come up while inhaling, then exhale and breathe normally.

CONCENTRATION: Upon the movements.

THERAPEUTIC RESULTS: It brings suppleness to the lumbar region, articulations of the knees, and ankles. It also massages the abdominal organs, and enhances the body's equilibrium.

Dr. Lauture Massac

OTHER VARIANTS OF MATSYENDRASANA

We already have seen this posture. However, in order to achieve easily the *Matsyendrasana*, one must practice regularly the variants, which are many. They are very useful, mostly for students with stiff legs.

FIRST VARIANT EXECUTION:

Sitting on the ground with straight legs, place the right leg upon the left thigh. The right leg is almost in a vertical position, and the right foot is flat on the floor between the left thigh and the knee. Turn carefully the trunk to the left side, and then pass the left arm upon and near the right knee. This knee should be kept, if possible, under the left armpit. The right arm is straight behind the back in the axis of the body with the hands flat on the floor near the pelvis. Press the right thigh against the abdomen by the pressure of the left arm, and then the left hand should remain flat on the floor. Keep rotating the trunk until the shoulders are in the same line. Hold on the posture a few seconds and then breathe normally. After some resting time, give it up and reverse the position.

This posture should be studied carefully. In most cases, if it is performed easily, that means it is done in the wrong way. Study the description, read it again and try to understand it better.

SECOND VARIANT EXECUTION:

To start, follow the description of the first variant, but in this one the left leg is bent instead of being straight. The left thigh is in the axis of the floor, the heel of the left foot is near the right buttock. Just as in the previous posture, pass the right leg upon the left thigh, and keep the right foot flat on the floor between the left thigh and the knee. Pass the left arm upon the right knee and catch the right foot with the left hand. After a few seconds, rotate the trunk to the right. The right arm is straight behind the back with the hands flat on the floor near the pelvis. Stress the rotation by placing the right thigh against the abdomen with a deep pressure of the left arm. Both shoulders should remain on the same line.

Keep the position as long as you can, and then breathe normally. After some rest, give it up and reverse the position.

SOME DIFFICULTIES: If you are unable to catch your foot with the hand of the opposite arm, then catch the knee which is flat on the floor to help maintain the posture. If you are losing your balance behind, it is probably because your right hand flat on the floor is too far from the pelvis. Watch for both of your shoulders, which should be at the same height and on the same axis.

CONCENTRATION: Upon the spinal column.

BREATHING: Slow and regular.

THERAPEUTIC RESULTS: This asana may help to rectify scoliosis of the spine and strengthen the lateral cords of the sympathetic system. It also massages the abdominal organs and improves the nervous system.

THE COW POSTURE (BHADRASANA)

From the standing position, sit down on the heels. Stay on the point of the toes, separate the legs and the thighs as much as possible. For that, take the help of the toes, which should be close to each other, and heel against heel. Keep the body erect. Bring both hands folded at the chest level, and then hold the posture as long as you can without swinging, and then breathe normally. After some time, come up slowly and repeat the exercise two or three times.

CONCENTRATION: Keep it upon the balance, which should be maintained as steadily as possible.

BREATHING: Normal and regular.

RESULTS: This posture brings suppleness to the articulations of the feet, the ankles, and the hips. It develops steadiness of balance, and it is excellent for concentration.

VARIANT: From this posture described above, keep both hands straight on the floor, take a deep breath, and then exhaling, bend the body forward while trying to bring the forehead near to the floor. Hold the position with empty lungs as long as you can, and then come up breathing normally.

RESULTS: It affects more the lumbar muscles, the spine, and the joints of the thighs.

PRANAYAMA - THE ALTERNATE BREATHING WITH RETENTION

This pranayama is performed in the same manner as the alternate one previously described. However, after the inhalation, stop the breath with full lungs as long as you can before exhaling through the other nostril. The length of the breath retention should be about six seconds in the beginning and as the body system is getting used to it, increase the duration to twelve seconds. After a long practice and according to your own ability, you may extend the length of the retention up to twenty-four seconds.

CONCENTRATION: The same as in the simple alternate breathing.

RESULTS: The same, but more powerful.

THE COOL WAVES PRANAYAMA (Shitali)

Sit in any comfortable posture, squeeze the teeth and separate a little bit the lips. First empty the lungs, and then draw the air strongly between the teeth. You should feel a cool sensation. When the lungs are completely filled up, close the lips and exhale rapidly through both nostrils.

Both inhalation and exhalation must be done strongly and quickly. Repeat the exercise six to twelve times at least.

CONCENTRATION: On the throat center.

RESULTS: The yogic scriptures say that this pranayama oxygenizes and refreshes the blood and quenches the thirst sensation.

CHAPTER VIII

LESSON 6   **PART 1**

YOGA AND THE SPINAL COLUMN

In the human complex, the spinal column plays a very essential role. It is "the life tree" from which all the nervous commands of the organs go through. It protects the prolonged medulla which is the extension of the encephalic. It permits the static and the movements of the head and the trunk. On both sides of its trajectory are situated the ganglions of the nervous sympathetic system which assure the distribution of the vital influx to different parts of the body, as well as the transmission of the sensory impressions to the brain.

In the view of yoga, the spine is very important. It is for this reason that most of the essential yoga postures deal with it. It plays a major role in the distribution of prana, which first goes through it in the nervous system before spreading in the endocrine glands and the organs.

Among the twelve basic asanas we already have taught, ten are dealing with the spinal cord. On a different level, we will study in the third part of this lesson the *chakras*, or psychic centers, which receive and distribute the cosmic energies through the spinal column. The chakras are not located in the physical body; they are energetic centers residing in different parts of the ethereal body.

In the first part of this lesson we will deal only with the spinal column according to the point of view of physiology and anatomy. Let us look at some basic well-known anatomic views: (Cramer, G.D. & Darby, S.A. 2013).

The spinal column is made of a stack of vertebrae, some of which are welded with each other. Those that are not welded are united by some fibro-cartilage tissue or inter-vertebral discs. Later on, we shall tell about the important role of the inter-somatic discs. From the bottom to the top, there are:

1-The coccyx formed with four small welded vertebras.

2-The sacrum, formed with five big welded vertebras, in which the mass is set in between the two iliac bones;

3-the non-welded lumbar vertebras;

4-the 12 dorsal vertebras, which support 12 pairs of ribs;

5-the 7 cervical vertebras including Atlas, the highest one, which supports the head.

N.B. The mobile vertebrae are numbered from top to bottom of C1, the first cervical, to L5, the fifth lumbar vertebra.

The spinal column on its trajectory has 3 essential curvatures. One cervical curvature convexes forward, another dorsal one extending backward, and the lumbar, which also convexes forward. The accentuation of those curvatures may lead to a cervical lordosis or dorsal kyphosis (exaggerated rounding of the back). The spinal column may also get deformed at certain circumstances and lead to scoliosis. All of those different pathological afflictions of the spine could be improved by the practice of yoga postures.

THE VERTEBRAE

It is not necessary for us to describe the type of each vertebra in this book. Let us simply say that their volume grows bigger from top to bottom. The cervical vertebrae are smaller than the lumbar. The first cervical vertebra, or Atlas, which supports the head, has the form of a ring. It is mobile around a pivot which represents the second cervical vertebra, the Axis.

The vertebra is made of a compact body, with two bows which limit the protuberant vertebral hole. The stack of vertebrae constitutes a hollow channel made of each superposed vertebral hole in which the spinal marrow goes through. On the apophyses and the blades are attached many ligaments and muscular tendons which keep the vertebrae strongly welded between themselves. The lateral part of the vertebra has a notch which forms the *conjugation hole,* from which the rachidian nerve comes out.

THE DISC

The disc is the principal media which unites two vertebral bodies. It is made of fibro-cartilage and has a gelatinous cell, which is used at the same time as a shock-absorber and a distributor of pressure. When the disc is cracked, the cell may come out and lead to a herniated disc. The regular practice of yoga maintains the vitality and the suppleness of the intervertebral discs, and may retard its advanced growth. It also makes supple the vertebral articulations and many ligaments, mostly the anterior and the posterior ones, which are considered to be the most important.

THE ATTACHED MUSCLES TO THE SPINAL COLUMN

The sacral-lumbar mass, which is attached to the sacrum of the lumbar spine, and the long dorsal, which goes up to the cervical vertebras, are the most important spinal muscles. The trapezius muscle, which we already have studied, is attached to the shoulder blade and the superior part of the spinal column. It plays a very important role in yoga, and it is responsible for *torticollis,* abnormal of the neck.

YOGA AND THE MOVEMENTS OF THE SPINAL COLUMN

The spinal column is animated by various different movements which permit the trunk and the head to move in several directions. We will attempt to explain what those movements are and to what extent the asanas are affecting them. We must emphasize that the breadth of those movements depends on the healthy state of the somatic discs. That is why it is important to practice regularly the basic yoga postures in order to maintain the vitality of the discs and ligaments.

THE FLEXION – It is the movement which permits the joints of the spinal column to move forward. The hinge joints, which include the elbows, the ankles, the knees, are affected by constant powerful movements.

THE EXTENSION – It is the inverted flexion movement which allows the spinal column to move backwards. Its amplitude is inferior to the one of the flexion movement. The extension movement may correct minor kyphosis dorsal defects. The asanas which allow the holistic maintenance of those movements are *Bhujangasana, Ushtrasana, Setvasana,* and *Sarvangasana.* All of those postures are excellent to correct and to prevent rounded back.

LATERAL INCLINATION – The lateral inclination is the movement from which the spinal column can move from right to left in the plane of the body. Usually the flexion is double in the asanas, which are concerned with those movements. The asanas are: all the 4 variants of *Konasana* and the third variant of *Janusirasana.*

THE ROTATION – The rotation is the movement from which the spinal column can move backward, to the right, and to the left without any lateral extension or inclination. In this movement, the discs are affected by a powerful distortion and are extended to the maximum. The asanas which are concerned with the rotation movement are those which twist the trunk, such as *Konasana* and its variants. The third posture of *Janusirasana* is essentially a vertebral torsion posture, which is one of the different variants of *Matsyendrasana*.

LESSON 6   PART 2
THE ASANAS

Before starting with the second part of this lesson, it is helpful to go backward and ask a few essential questions about all you have studied during the past three months.

FIRST QUESTION: Are you performing correctly and slowly the asanas you have learned? It is suggested that you read the description of the postures again. You may have missed a detail which, in this reading, may attract your attention.

For example, in the tree posture (*Vrikshasana*), watch the body, which should be kept straight. Do not bend it to the right or to the left. Keep the folded leg perpendicular to the body. In the posterior stretch posture *Pascimottanasana*, do not lift the knees up. In the angle posture Konasana, the arms should be vertical and alongside of each other, and do not bend the knees. In the cobra posture (*Bhujangasana*), keep the feet close together. The arms should be straight, with the head bent backward. In the bow posture (*Dhanushasana*), watch not to separate the knees too much. In *Sarvangasana*, the body should be kept vertical, and avoid bending the back. If possible, let someone else check it for you. In *Matsyendrasana*, make sure that the arm is in the right place near the knee.

SECOND QUESTION: Are you sure that you are breathing correctly with the movement of the respiratory rhythm when it is indicated?

Each posture goes with its own way of breathing. Have you forgotten this? If so, then it is time to review the correct description given with the posture. You should keep in mind to synchronize the movement with the breathing. It is very important.

THIRD QUESTION: After each difficult posture or series of two to three postures which could exert much stress upon the body, are you resting in *Shavasana* for a few minutes? You should also remember to rest in *Shavasana* doing pranayama in order to store prana in the body.

FOURTH QUESTIONS: Are you practicing concentration with the asanas, as indicated on a particular part of the body?

STUDENT DAILY SESSION

Let us see now how you could adjust your yoga sessions. It depends, of course, on how much time you can arrange for that. A suggested session of 30 minutes, with 10 minutes for the practice of pranayama, should be reasonable. If you can budget more time, a full session of one hour should be plenty. Remember, it is not necessary to do too many asanas in one session, especially during your first six months of yoga practice. One should not hurry to master any posture. The mastery over a posture will automatically come over time. Too much stress upon the muscles and the nerves may hurt instead of doing any good. Be careful with the length of the retention of the breath. Let us recap the essential basic postures which you have learned up to now.

ESSENTIAL BASIC POSTURES

The full resting posture *Shavasana*
Salute to the sun *Surya Namaskar*
Posterior-stretch posture *Pascimottanasana*
Worship posture *Bhunamanavajrasana*
Tree posture *Vrikshasana*
Bow posture *Dhanushasana*
Swastika posture *Swastikasana*
Plough posture *Halasana*
Cobra posture *Bhujangasana*
Goraksa posture *Goraksasana*
Whole body posture *Sarvangasana*
Torsion posture *Matsyendrasana*

You may add *Uddiyana-banda Mudra*, which will be studied in the next lesson. It is not classified with the asanas, but instead with the *Kriyas* and *bandhas* (gestures for internal purification). It is also the same for the great prayer posture or *Bhunamanavajrasana*, which is also a Mudra (symbolic gesture).

We will also study in the seventh lesson the dolphin posture, which is also an essential posture. It will replace the complete *shirs-Asana*, which we do not advise you to try without the presence of a well-trained teacher.

If you only can budget ten minutes a day for yoga practice, this is our recommendation:

First practice *Surya Namaskar* (salutation to the sun) three times. Sit in *Swastika* or *Sukhasana* for the practice of pranayama. Practice six *Kumbhaka Pranayama* (with breath retention), and six alternate ones. Then practice the whole-body posture *Sarvangasana* one time and hold the position for approximately one minute. Continue with the plough posture *Halasana* one time for about one minute, and then do the resting posture *Shavasana* for one minute. Follow up with the posterior stretch posture *Pascimottanasana*, and alternate on each side. Do the cobra posture, *Bhujangasana*, three times, and finally end with *Shavasana*, the full resting posture, for approximately two minutes. This series of postures are sufficient to keep you in good condition for the whole day.

Now we suggest that for this week to try to improve *Sarvangasana* and its variants with the vertebral torsion posture. For the study and the improvement of a difficult yoga posture, try to do them outside of your regular yoga session. A regular yoga session should be well synchronized and in harmony with that peaceful state of mind we have described in the first lesson, in order to attract positive cosmic energies into the body. Always remember the positive effects of the creative power of thoughts. Mental concentration increases the effectiveness of pranayama. The concentration upon the respiratory rhythm should be done especially in the sitting postures. While performing the asanas, the mental concentration should be focused upon the movements which lead to the posture and upon those leading back to the starting position.

At the same time, it should also be directed upon the breathing. It is better to first perform all the standing postures, and then proceed to those lying on the back. Next execute the sitting ones and then finish with the postures performed while lying on the belly. Remember to switch over to one starting position, and then to another starting position with the same slow speed, which should also be observed in the execution of the asanas.

THE ANGLE POSTURE (Konasana Variant)

EXECUTION: Standing up, separate the legs and cross the arms behind the back. Take a deep breath, and slowly incline to the right while trying to touch the knee with the forehead. Hold the breath and stay in the posture a few seconds; come back up inhaling and then exhale. Do the same movements to the left side, and then repeat the exercise three times from each side.

CONCENTRATION: Upon the respiratory rhythm.

BREATHING: As it is described in the exercise.

THERAPEUTIC RESULTS: This posture brings suppleness to the spinal column and rejuvenates the lymphatic system. It reduces fatness upon the hips; prevents and improves cellulitis of the abdomen. It also lengthens the dorsal lateral muscles and strengthens the abdominal muscles.

A VARIANT OF THE TREE POSTURE (Vrikshasana)

From the first tree posture described in the third lesson, which you should know how to perform, do this variant.

EXECUTION: In this tree posture, with foot upon the thigh, cross the hands behind the nape of the neck, and bend the bust slowly forward, while trying to maintain your balance. Keep the position as long as you can with empty lungs, and come back up with the inhalation. Reverse the position of the foot and repeat the exercise 2 to 3 times on each side.

BREATHING: As indicated in the exercise.

CONCENTRATION: Upon the balance of the posture.

RESULTS: The same as in the first tree posture, but it increases the sense of physical equilibrium.

DANCE POSTURE (Nrityasana)

EXECUTION: Stand up and breathe normally. Concentrate first on the balance of the body, and then slowly bend the right leg backward and then catch the big toes. Raise the left hand up and try to maintain your balance. The bust should remain as straight as possible. After some time, reverse the position.

BREATHING: Slow and regular.

CONCENTRATION: Upon the balance of the posture.

RESULTS: It makes the hip articulations supple, strengthens the intercostal muscles, and develops the sense of physical balance.

JANUSIR POSTURE (Janusirasana)
POSTURE 1

EXECUTION: From the student posture already studied, sit with the left leg straight and the right one folded near the thigh, and keep the bust straight. While inhaling, raise both arms in a vertical position. Bend the bust forward while exhaling, and then keep the arms straight until they can catch the left foot. If you can, keep the forehead on the knee as long as you can, and then hold your breath. Come back up, inhale, and reverse the position of the leg. Repeat this posture three to four times from each side.

CONCENTRATION: Upon the solar plexus.

BREATHING: As described in the posture.

RESULTS: It develops the back muscles, prevents and reduces fatness on the hips, makes supple the muscles of the legs and the thighs.

POSTURE 2

EXECUTION: Take the same starting position of the student posture. Sit with the left leg straight and the right one folded near the thigh. Bend down and catch the ankles of the left leg with both hands, and then slowly lift up the left leg. Keep it straight up and help yourself only with the arms. Keep rising up the leg without bending forward and try to touch your forehead with the knee. Stay in the position as long as you can, with the right knee remaining flat on the floor, and then breathe normally. After some time, reverse the position.

BREATHING: Regular and normal.

CONCENTRATION: Upon the position.

RESULTS: It makes supple the articulations of the hips and the legs.

THE PERFECT POSTURE (Siddhasana)

Since this posture is more comfortable than the lotus one for meditation, you should try to master it as soon as possible.

EXECUTION: Sit on the floor, fold the right leg with the heel near the scrotum region. Catch the left leg and place it upon the right one. Both knees should be on the floor, and keep straight the spinal column. Keep both hands relaxed on the knees. Breathe normally and remain in the posture as long as you can to develop the strength of the spine and resistance of the legs and the knees.

MENTAL CONCENTRATION: Upon the heart region

RESULTS: This is one of the best postures for the practice of pranayama, concentration, and meditation. It rectifies the defects of the spine and acts upon the equilibrium of the nervous system.

A THIRD VARIANT OF SARVANGASANA

EXECUTION: From the second variant of *Sarvangasana* or the whole-body posture, instead of taking the support of your arms flat on the floor, you keep them on a vertical position alongside the thighs. The whole body is resting upon the head and the shoulders. Stay in the posture as long as you can, and then after some time keep the hands on the floor and slowly bring the trunk down, and then take rest in *Shavasana.*

MENTAL CONCENTRATION: Upon the heart region.

BREATHING: Regular.

RESULTS: The same as in those two other variants described before. It also acts upon the balance of the physical body.

HALF LOCUST POSTURE (Ardhashalabhasana)

Lie on the belly, the arms straight alongside the body with the hands flat on the floor. Lift the right leg straight up and keep it as high as possible while inhaling. Keep it there a few seconds and lower the leg down while exhaling. Do the same thing with the other leg. Finally, repeat the exercise three to four times with each leg.

CONCENTRATION: Upon the lumbar region.

BREATHING: As described with the posture.

THERAPEUTIC RESULTS: It strengthens the lumbar region, helps with constipation, purifies the kidneys, and irrigates the lungs with fresh blood.

THE SCIENCE OF BREATHING (Pranayama)
MANIPUR MUDRA PRANAYAMA

EXECUTION: Sit down in any comfortable posture and completely empty the lungs. Take a deep, strong inhalation through both nostrils and stop the breath for a few seconds, and then with a sudden contraction of the abdominal muscles, push the belly out. Keep the position as long as you can, and then strongly blow the air out through the nostrils. Take another abdominal inhalation and repeat the exercise between six and twelve times.

CONCENTRATION: On the coming and going of the flow of the air.

RESULTS: It is supposed to purify the nostril passage, the throat center, and the lungs.

THE ALTERNATE PRANAYAMA (Surya-Bheda,
or The Splitting Sun)

EXECUTION: Sit down in any comfortable posture; use the thumb and the two last fingers of the right hand to block the passage of the air in the nostrils. You already know the technique of alternate pranayama; you have been practicing since the fourth lesson. The rhythmical alternate pranayama has the same basic principal. The only difference is that inhalation, exhalation, and retention are performed according to different length of time in the rhythm. For this pranayama, the recommended rhythm is: 4-16-8. Inhalation: 4 seconds – Retentions: 16 seconds – Exhalation: 8 seconds.

CONCENTRATION: Upon the pranayama.

RESULTS: It purifies the nostril conduits, reacts upon the nervous system, and prepares the mind for meditation.

༄

LESSON 6   **PART 3**
HIGHER YOGA
The Energy Receptors
And Distribution Centers (Chakras)

In the previous lesson, we emphasized the essential role of the ethereal body of humans, the Microcosm.

We will now study the power center, or *Chakras*, which receive and distribute the energy. In the human ethereal body, different energies are flowing in several impact points situated around its belt. Those focal points have different names. In the yogic terminology, they are called *Chakras,* or *Lotus Points.* According to Westerners, they are known as psychic centers.

The psychic centers in humans are many. It is not necessary to know them all. The yogic science revealed to us 72,000 *nadis*, or psychic nerve centers. However, the yoga Shastras deal only with seven main ones (Satchidananda, S. 1978).

It must be understood that the yogic science does not locate the seven main chakras in the gross physical body. They are rather characterized as psychic centers in the ethereal body. When those psychic centers are fully developed, the yogi obtains mastery over the body. Here are the names and locations of those psychic centers:

At the bottom of the spinal column near the sacrum region is situated the *Muladhar Chakra.*

In the lumbar region is situated the *Swadhistan Chakra.*

At the naval region is situated the *Manipur Chakra.*

At the heart center is the location of *Anahat Chakra.*

At the throat center is the location of *Vishuddha Chakra.*

At the center between the eyebrows is the location of *Ajna Chakra.*

At the top of the head, the crown center is the location of *Sahasrara Chakra* or *Brahmaranda.*

In the yogic terminology the chakras are associated with the shape of a lotus. In fact, colors and petals correspond to the quality of the energies which flow in the centers. It is important to know that the chakras are not awakened by flowing energies. Their vitality depends on the spiritual evaluative degree of the person. According to each spiritual stage reached, the particular chakra corresponding to that spiritual stage is awakened and starts sending vibrations to its center at a rhythm which becomes faster and faster. It then becomes receptive to the energy that is flowing in it. In other cases, the chakra remains sleeping and is not synchronized with the vibrating energy that could animate it. The area of the body which is controlled by it remains in a lethargic state.

In the body of the highly spiritually developed human, all the psychic centers are vibrating at a reasonable rate. In other human beings, certain centers are still asleep, with some having just awakened, and some others already fully active.

In the body of a highly developed yogi, all the chakras are vibrating with the cosmic energies. That is why all the organs of the physical body are well supplied with vitality and the result is a perfect physical and mental health. It is through this perfect physical and mental harmony that the regular practice of higher yoga will lead.

RELATIONSHIP BETWEEN THE CENTERS

Each lower center is connected with a higher center corresponding with it. The Muladhar center is connected with the Sahasrara. Those two centers (chakras) play a major role in the self-realization concept. We shall explain this in another lesson.

The Swadhistan center is related to Vishuddha center. During the process of spiritual development, the yogi controls the pranic energy up to the throat center. The yogi then becomes a creator on higher level.

The navel region (Manipur center), which is the emotional center where all gross energies are discharged for transmutation, is related to the Anahat center. The difficult task for the yogis is to bring up the powerful energies which are discharged in the Manipur center to the Anahat center.

For that to happen, one must first transform emotional physical desires into higher, universal spiritual desires. This is still the prerogative of few dedicated gifted sadhakas. However, as universal karma is moving toward purification, it will become the apanage of the whole humanity.

This particular relationship between the lower centers and the higher centers should not remove in our mind the fact that all the centers are connected with each other. For example, the Shahasrara center is directing all the other centers. Concerning the Ajna center—from a certain stage of spiritual achievement, it becomes a synthesis center.

The centers are interconnected by some channels, or energy wires that are more important than the energy wires that formed the nadis. The substance which formed those ethereal channels comes from the planetary prana. We will study prana and the nadis in the next lesson.

We need to keep in mind that in yogic literatures, the nadis, or pranic tubes, convey all the energies, no matter what level they come from, according to the degree of spiritual evolution of each person. The seven major centers vibrate to the energies of the seven life rays of the solar system. However, this could be true only for the well-developed yogis. In most cases, some energies coming from the solar source go through the centers without vibrating them and without shaking up the sleeping chakras.

As soon as the chakras are pierced and animated by the power of the *pranic kundalini*, the sadhaka becomes a spiritually awakened human being. At this point, many conscious spheres with greater areas of transcendental knowledge are accessible. The process of evolution is developing life after life, until the day when the coronal center at the top of the head (Sahasrara chakra) will at last manifest the glory of a realized human being.

CHAPTER IX

YOGA AND THE RESPIRATORY SYSTEM

In the science of yoga, the respiratory system plays a very important role. You have now become familiar with the science of breathing, and you know how prana is distributed in the cells of the body. The prana which is collected through the control of pranayama is carried away by the blood and the nervous system. The prana is the vital energy of the planetary system in which every living being is bathed. Without prana, life cannot be. However, prana cannot be identified or compared with atmospheric oxygen. It is considered as an electro-magnetic energy more subtler than the chemical component of the air, which is known to science.

In this chapter, we will deal with the respiratory system according to the actual anatomical and physiological datum. However, we will not forget to talk about prana, this electro-magnetic energy which science has not yet discovered. It can be understood only through the practice of yoga. If you practice regularly the science of yoga, you will soon experience prana within your own self. Now, let us study briefly the anatomy and the physiological aspect of the respiratory system, which is very important to know in the practice of yoga.

THE ORGANS AND THE TRACKS
OF THE RESPIRATION

The respiratory organs open on the exterior middle by the nose. In the practice of yoga, it is emphasized that one should breathe through the nose and not through the mouth, because the nasal fossae warm up the air and prevent dust from entering the respiratory system.

In the yogic point of view, the equilibrium of pranic current depends on the proper maintenance of the nasal fossae. This justifies the importance of alternate practice of pranayama. After the nasal fossae, we find the pharynx and the larynx (vocal organs), then the trachea, which is a tube supported by some cartilaginous rings. The trachea artery is divided in two bronchia. Both bronchia are connected with the lungs.

THE LUNGS

The lungs consist of two sponging elastic masses situated in the thoracic cage. The right lung has three lobes and the left one only two. The hilum forms the totality of the lung, where all the bronchia and the blood vessels are penetrating. The lung is surrounded and protected by a membrane called the pleura (Emery, J. 2014).

The lungs are joined at the thoracic cage by the pleura. It is the movements of the thoracic cage which draws those of the lungs. The movements of the thoracic cage are released by the respiratory muscles, of which the most important one is the diaphragm muscle, already studied in previous lessons.

DURING INHALATION: In the complete yogic breathing, the components of abdominal, median, and superior breathing are acting successively with the diaphragm, the elevating muscles of the ribs, the pectoral, and the scalene muscles.

DURING EXHALATION: The same muscles are loosened. The transversus abdominal muscles, when hollow to the maximum, allow the maximum raising up movement of the diaphragm and the expelling of polluted air from the lungs

Breathing is an act which can be voluntarily put under control of the willpower. It is through breath control that the yogis come to master their internal organs. However, ordinary natural breathing is totally independent from the will; during sleep, it is working automatically. Automatic breathing is a reflex movement. Most people, with the exception of advanced yogis, breathe unconsciously. Complete inhalation and complete exhalation are performed during the practice of pranayama.

THE PULMONARY CAPACITY

It is interesting for the yoga students to have a little knowledge about this subject. In normal unconscious breathing, we inhale and exhale about 1.5 liters of current air. In the complete yogic breathing, we inhale and exhale about 3.5 liters of air, which is about seven times more in volume than in unconscious breathing. From this comes the essential interest of the completely controlled yogic breathing to maintain health and vitality of the organism. After a complete yogic exhalation, 1.5 liters of air remain in the lungs. It is this remaining air which allows the retention of the breath with empty lungs. The residual air in the lungs will assure the oxygenation of the blood.

THE RELATIONSHIP BETWEEN THE RESPIRATORY SYSTEM AND THE CIRCULATORY SYSTEM IN YOGA

A detailed study of those relationships will go beyond the frame of this book. We will only point out a few essential remarks. We distinguish two circulations: the general circulation or the big one, and the pulmonary circulation or the small one. Both are bound together and go through the heart, the central organ of the circulatory system. The ancient sages were well aware of the relationship between the respiratory system and the circulatory system. The rhythmical contraction of the heart is not under the control of the willpower. However, a trained advanced yogi is able to slow or accelerate the rhythms of the heart by controlling the respiratory activity. This is one of the goals of the yogic science of pranayama. After a complete session of pranayama we can ascertain that the pulsation numbers have diminished. It is the same in breath retention with full lungs, and we can feel the immediate slowdown of the heart rhythm.

At the institute of yoga at Lonavala near Mumbai (India), or elsewhere in the world, many scientific tests have been conducted on the yogis to detect the claims of yoga therapy on the human body. The electrocardiogram has shown the truthfulness of yogic actions on the body.

The goal for ordinary people is not to reach this yogic perfection. However, it is good to know that in this field it is possible to obtain positive results with the practice of yoga. With this knowledge, one should be more encouraged in practicing yoga.

ॐ

LESSON 7   **PART 2**

THE ASANAS

TREE LIFT-UP POSTURE (Utthita-Vrikshasana)
EXECUTION: Standing up, lift up your right foot to the knee. Catch it in this way: with the right hand taking the point and the left hand taking

the heel; and then, with the help of both hands, lift up the right foot slowly as high as possible, while maintaining the balance on the left leg. In the beginning, you may find it difficult to keep the balance. You should not bend the body forward or bend the left knee. By practicing, one day you may be able raise the foot up to the throat center or the chin. Hold on to the posture as long as possible, and then bring the foot back down slowly and reverse the position of the legs.

CONCENTRATION: Upon the physical and mental balance.

RESPIRATION: It should be slow and superficial.

RESULTS: It is excellent for the physical and mental balance. It brings suppleness to the knee joints, and acts upon the abdominal glands and organs.

THE FEET STRETCH POSTURE (Kandapidanasana)

EXECUTION: Sit on the ground; place the feet together, heels against each other, just as in *Goraksasana*. Catch the feet together with both hands. Press the feet continuously and slowly, and then try to bring them near the abdomen, while raising them up as high as possible without losing your balance. The thighs are separated to the maximum. Hold on to the position as long as you can. Keep the bust erect, breathe normally, and after some time, bend the legs forward and take a rest. Repeat the posture three to four times.

CONCENTRATION: Upon the muscles of the thigh.

RESPIRATION: Regular.

RESULTS: It brings suppleness to the articulations of the knees, the thighs, and the hips.

POWERFUL LEGS POSTURE (Pada-Ugrasana)

To master this posture completely requires a long practice of all other leg asanas.

EXECUTION: Sit on the ground, separate the straight legs as much as possible. Bend the bust forward and then try to bring the forehead down as near as possible to the ground. Catch the toes with the straight arms.

In the beginning, it may not be possible for you to catch the toes, so just keep the hands on the legs.

CONCENTRATION: Upon the solar plexus.

RESPIRATION: First, inhale and then exhale while bending; keep the posture and hold on to the breath with empty lungs. Inhale while coming back up, and then exhale. Second, while performing the posture you may also breathe normally.

RESULTS: It gives suppleness to the spinal column and the internal upward muscles of the thighs. It massages the area of the thyroid gland, rejuvenates the nervous system, and increases the digestive power.

A VARIANT OF THE PLOUGH POSTURE (Halasana)
EXECUTION: From the *Halasana* posture you already have studied, stretch farther upon the flexion of the trunk, and keep the legs and the feet straight. Instead of placing the arms flat on the floor, bend them and place the hands behind the head.

RESPIRATION: Abdominal.

CONCENTRATION: Upon the thyroid gland.

RESULTS: The pressure on the throat is more powerful. The thyroid gland is irrigated by fresh blood, and the spine becomes more flexible.

THE WHEEL POSTURE (Chakra Asana)
EXECUTION: Kneeling on the floor, bend the trunk backward. Catch the ankles with the hands while keeping the head bent as much as possible, and then keep the arms straight. Maintain the posture as long as possible, and then come back slowly and bend forwards with the forehead on the floor.

CONCENTRATION: Upon the region of the thyroid gland.

RESPIRATION: Slow and regular.

RESULTS: It makes the spinal column more flexible, and acts upon the kidneys. It strengthens and tightens the abdominal muscles and exerts a powerful action upon the windpipe (trachea and the larynx).

THE DOLPHIN POSTURE (Matsyabhedanasana)

This posture is considered to be the first to the achievement of the complete *Shirshasana* or the headstand posture. By starting with this posture, you will get almost the same therapeutic effects of the full headstand position. For those of you who feel ready to attempt the full headstand posture, first start practicing behind a wall to avoid falling.

EXECUTION: Kneeling on the floor, interlace the fingers of both hands, and then place the head in the middle of the interlaced hands, which now comes behind the nape of the head. The elbows and the forearms are resting on the floor. Lift up the knees and walk slowly towards the elbows and go as far as you can. When you have reached where you cannot move any farther toward the elbows, you need to hold on to the position as long as you can. To attempt a full headstand, raise one leg up, which should be followed by the other.

CONCENTRATION: On the head.

RESPIRATION: Just follow your breathing

RESULTS: This asana irrigates the brain, the pineal, and the pituitary glands with fresh blood. It increases memory power and cerebral capacity.

EXERCISES FOR INTERNAL PURIFICATION (Kriyas)

Those internal purification exercises are classified in yogic literature between the asanas and the breathing. Their roles are to massage the internal organs of the abdominal and to invigorate the viscera.

ABDOMINAL RETRACTION (Uddiyan-Bandha Mudra)
EXERCISE 1
EXECUTION: Standing up, separate the legs a little bit, and then place the hands flat on the thighs. Inhale thoroughly, and then exhale completely the air from the lungs, hold on the breath and incline the trunk forwards. While stopping the breath, contract the abdomen inward as much as you can. The abdominal wall should come as close as possible to the lumbar spine. Keep the contraction for a few seconds and then come back to the initial position and breathe normally.

OBSERVATION:

1-Before contracting in the abdomen to the maximum, the air must be exhaled completely and the diaphragm raised-up.

2-By pressing the hands tightly upon the thighs, you can increase the abdominal contraction.

CONCENTRATION: Upon the exercise.

RESULTS: It gives a powerful massage to the cavity of the abdominal organs, purifies and invigorates the viscera. Practice the exercise between 3 and 6 times.

EXERCISE 2: RAISING UP THE ABDOMEN.

This second Kriya has a more powerful effect upon the superior organs of the abdominal cavity. For the previous one especially, it affects the interior organs of the cavity.

EXECUTION: Standing up with closed feet, inhale deeply. Place hands, palms, and fingers against each other and exhale slowly. At the end of the inhalation, contract the abdominal muscles from bottom to top, while raising up the diaphragm. Hold the air a few seconds, and then inhale slowly and breathe normally. Repeat this exercise between three and six times.

OBSERVATION: By pressing both hands tightly against each other, the possibility of contraction is increased.

CONCENTRATION: Upon the exercise.

RESULTS: Same results as in the previous exercise.

ADVICE: Those two Kriyas, if they are performed in the right way, have a tremendous beneficial effect upon the abdominal organs. Start practicing each exercise once and progressively increase the number of attempts.

THROAT CONTRACTION (Jalandhara-Bandha)

This exercise is also considered to be a *Kriya*. It can be performed in a standing or sitting position. We will describe it in the sitting position.

EXECUTION: Sit in any comfortable posture. Take a deep inhalation, and then slowly bend the head forward and exhale. The chin is pressed tightly against the throat region. Hold the contraction along with the breath as long as you can, and then raise the head back up while inhaling, and finally breathe normally.

OBSERVATION: You may increase the contraction by pressing the hands tightly on the knees.

CONCENTRATION: Upon the throat center (Vishuddha chakra).

RESULTS: Invigorates the thyroid glands, ventilates the lungs completely, and purifies the median passages of the respiratory system.

THE SCIENCE OF BREATHING (Pranayama)
AND THE STIMULUS BREATHING (Ujayi Pranayama)

EXECUTION: Take any comfortable sitting posture. First, empty completely the lungs and inhale through both nostrils for approximately 8 seconds. Hold on the breath for 8 seconds, and then exhale through the mouth for 16 seconds while making a whistle sound. To start with another round, empty the lungs completely.

REMARKS: In the beginning, it might be difficult to inhale for 8 seconds. You can start inhaling slowly in order for the lungs not to get filled-up before the 8 seconds.

RESULTS: It stimulates the endocrine glands.

THE ALTERNATE PURIFICATION BREATHING

By now, we assume that you are quite knowledgeable about the correct performance of the simple purification breathing. Concerning the alternate breathing, it is quite easy to perform.

EXECUTION: Inhale completely through both nostrils, and then stop the breath a few seconds while pushing the belly out. Close the right nostril and exhale the air in one blow through the left nostril, and inhale again through both nostrils. Close the left one and exhale through the right nostril. Alternate the nostril only for the exhalation. To finish, repeat this exercise three times in each nostril.

CONCENTRATION: This pranayama will purify the nostril tracks, the throat, and the lungs. After many pranayama exercises, you must take rest in *Shavasana* to allow the storing prana to spread itself all over the organs.

❧

LESSON 7   PART 3
HIGHER YOGA
The Vital Energy of the Prana

This is the time to deal more in-depth with prana, the cosmic manifested energy. Most of the important therapeutic results of yoga are attributed to pranic energy.

Prana is itself the cosmic life and accordingly the life of the human, whose being is in the vital cosmic body. Prana is the energy which nourishes and sustains the human microcosm of life. It can be compared with the third aspect of the divine energy, which is the divine energy of the Holy Spirit of Brahma.

However, if one receives prana from the planetary sources, the planet itself receives it from the sun, and the sun receives it from a vaster cosmic complex. Here, just as in the whole creation, we can understand it from the great cosmological corresponding law: "What is above is just like what is below; and what is below is just like what is above."

We should not think that there is only one manifestation of prana. If the prana is in fact ONE ENERGY, it must exist at different levels which correspond to different levels of the creation. Prana is manifested in the human body through the seven centers, or chakras, to develop the ethereal or vital body.

The human being nourishes life in the body with prana and the physical body itself with food. From this comes the interest of proper food in the body. The prana also enters the body through yogic breathing or pranayama exercises and proper diet. Besides those two ways to attract prana in the body, the yogi gets access to the more subtle aspects of it through meditation. The awakening of the psychic centers permits the yogi to develop tremendously the ethereal body, which is permanently bathed in the cosmic prana. The practice of higher yoga will draw higher vibrating energies to the yogi and will accelerate the spiritual evolution and assure the physical health of the body.

We have specified that prana is manifested in the vital or ethereal body through the seven chakras. It is conducted in the ethereal body by the nadis, which are considered as energy wires. The nadis are the subtractive parts of the nervous system, and transmit to it the vital energy which becomes the nervous influx. Millions and millions of nadis form millions and millions of nervous ramifications. The nadis intersect particularly in the surrounding of the plexus, but they are not considered to be those material plexuses. The tighter the nadis's wires are, the more the pranic current can freely circulate. The nervous system becomes well-balanced, resistant, and the physical health is strengthened.

CHAPTER X

THE DIGESTIVE SYSTEM

I n hatha yoga, the digestive system occupies the most important place. The health of the whole body complex depends upon the digestive process. In this chapter, we will study the role of the digestive organs.

1-THE DIGESTIVE SYSTEM:

Digestion is done by the alimentary canal. In the yogic literature, it is also well-known that digestion starts in the mouth and ends in the anus. That is why the yogis advised to eat slowly and grind well the food in the mouth before swallowing. The whole alimentary canal is lined with mucous membranes. Within these lines are countless number of small glands secreting digestive fermented juices or enzymes.

2-FIRST PROCESS OF DIGESTION:

The first part of digestion in the mouth is the mechanical reduction of the food into fine particles so that the digestive juices can act upon every particle of food. As the work of the teeth is going on, aided by the tongue, the food gets mixed with saliva, which provides the medium for chemical digestion. Saliva is secreted by special glands situated in different parts of the mouth. The flow of saliva is induced by reflex actions such as smell, sight, thought, hunger, etc. Between meals, only enough saliva is secreted to keep the mouth wet. The main ferment or enzyme that is present in saliva is ptyalin. This acts only on starch in the food, converting it into sugar.

If the saliva glands are not working properly, the first part of the digestion is not performed properly. Many yoga asanas, mostly those affecting the thyroid gland, will help the saliva glands to perform their duty and to send the digested food into the stomach for the next process (Bess-Boss, A., & Edelberg, D. 2009).

3-STOMACH DIGESTION:

The stomach is the most dilated portion of the whole alimentary canal. It lies in the upper part of the abdomen, just below the diaphragm. The stomach is just below the heart with the diaphragm in between the two. It is for this reason that when a condition of flatulence (wind formation) is created in the stomach, the space available for the heart to function becomes limited and a condition of palpitation may set up. The practice of yoga asanas may prevent or alleviate such organic condition.

The stomach is a highly muscular and elastic bag in herbivorous animals; that is why it is capable of doing a lot of grinding. In adult human beings, it can yield to a capacity of 3 to 5 pints. This is, of course, on the high side. But allowing it to enlarge to its maximum capacity is not to the advantage of the eater; this will mean eating tomorrow's food today. Persisting in that habit, one will have to miss several tomorrows and thus shorten one's life. The pyloric sphincter prevents a quick passing down into the small intestines of food until the food has been sufficiently digested.

An empty stomach is contracted, and its membranes are thrown into folds. As the food descends into the stomach, passing through cardiac sphincter, gentle movements begin. Waves of contraction move from the fundus, or the broad end, down to the pyloric, or the narrow end. Successive waves occur at intervals of about 20 seconds. Food is disintegrated and well-mixed with gastric juice. After sufficient time of wave movements, the pyloric sphincter relaxes to allow small quantities of digested food to enter the first part of the intestines known as the duodenum, but no solid will be allowed to pass through. If by mistake a solid piece passes down, the sphincter suddenly constricts and causes a stomach ache. This could become more unlikely if mastication is thorough and if regular asanas are practiced. Different kinds of food need different lengths of time to be digested. For example, a light vegetarian meal may take between 2 and 3 hours to be digested, while a heavy meal with plenty of meat may take longer to do the same job. Such a lengthy digesting process may stress out the internal organ by increasing their working duty, and therefore may contribute to the premature aging process of the body.

a) THE DUODENUM – The first part of the small intestines, which is approximately 10 inches, is called the *duodenum*. This is of very great importance in the digestive journey. It is in this part that the duct from the liver, after combining with the duct from the pancreas, joins the main alimentary canal. The food enters this part in an almost liquefied state, called the chyme.

b) THE PANCREAS – The pancreas is a narrow, longish glandular organ lying behind the lower edge of the stomach. Its duct unites with that of the liver and joins the duodenum about 3 inches below the pyloric sphincter. The pancreas has two kinds of secretions, external and internal.

The external secretions are the ones that pour into the duodenum along with the secretions of the liver. The internal secretion is insulin, which is helpful in the metabolism of carbohydrates.

c) THE LIVER – The liver is the largest glandular organ in the body. It has two large sections, called the right and the left lobes. The main job of the liver is to filter the blood flowing to the digestive track before it spreads to the rest of the body. Attached to the under-surface of the liver is a small storage for the bile called the *gall bladder*. Sometimes stones could develop in the gall bladder, and if they are not able to pass naturally through urine, medical intervention is needed to remove them. It is known that regular yoga asanas that massage the area of the liver could help in the prevention of gall bladder stones.

4-THE SMALL INTESTINE:

The small intestine is the continuous part of the duodenum. It is small in cross section, but has a very long way to carry the food for digestive purposes. Its length is approximately 22 feet. It is here that absorption starts. Digested fats, as an alkaline milky fluid, pass from the small intestine through the lymphatic system and then to the blood stream, and finally end up in a single channel called the thoracic duct.

In spite of the fact that the secretions in the stomach and the intestine are acidic, the digestive organs always remain alive and are not affected by the acids. However, when the acidic concentration increases and there is no food matter to act upon the digestive system, the intestine or the stomach becomes a prey to the acids. The regular practice of yoga asanas and pranayama strengthen the abdominal muscles, purify the blood, and therefore may reduce stomach acidity.

The intestines are in constant motion for mixing and for propulsion. The presence of food by itself provides the stimulus for this propulsive activity. The rate of peristalsis is about one inch in a minute. So it takes approximately six hours for the first part of the food to reach the end of the small intestine, although it is not considered to be the end of digestion. The rest of the matter has to move, and the whole matter has also to traverse the large intestine.

5-THE LARGE INTESTINE:

The entrance of the large intestine is guarded by a special band of muscles known as the *sphincter muscles valve* which separate the small intestine from the large intestine. Its function is to limit the flow-back of colonic contents into the ileum or the final section of the small intestine.

In yoga we consider the intestines as the large motors within the factory of the stomach. It is there where all chemical processes take place to keep the entire body functioning. That is why the quality of food intake is important to assure proper digestion and maintenance of healthy organs within the system. The goal of yoga is to maintain a healthy body with a healthy mind.

∾

LESSON 8   **PART 2**
THE ASANAS
The Great Symbolic Gesture (Maha Mudra)
This posture with its variants is also called a *Mudra*, because of its esoteric aspects.

FIRST POSTURE

EXECUTION: Sit on the floor with both legs straight. Bend the right leg and place the foot near the perineum with the other leg remaining straight. Place both hands on the floor near the knees with the bust erect. Take a deep inhalation and slowly bend the bust forward as much as you can. The head is down with the chin pressing on the chest. Hold the position with empty lungs a few seconds and then come back up, while inhaling. Repeat the exercise three to six times on each side, after reversing the leg position.

CONCENTRATION: Upon the throat center

RESULTS: It strengthens the back and the neck muscles, reinvigorates the thyroid gland, and gives suppleness to the legs and the thigh muscles.

RESPIRATION: As indicated in the posture.

SECOND POSTURE (Variant)

EXECUTION: Sit in the same position as in the previous asana with straight legs. Bend the left leg near the perineum, and keep the right leg straight. Take a deep inhalation and bend the bust forward. Catch the right foot and encircle it with both hands. Hold the position with empty lung for a few seconds, and come back up while inhaling and reverse the position of the legs. Repeat the exercise three to six times on each side.

CONCENTRATION: Upon the thyroid gland.

RESPIRATION: As indicated with the asana, but in order to hold the posture a little bit longer you may give up the retention and breathe normally.

RESULTS: Same as in the first posture, but increases the effects on spinal column.

COMPLETE LOCUST POSTURE (Purnashalabhasana)

EXECUTION: Lay with the belly flat on the floor, with the feet close to each other and the arms straight alongside the body. Make a fist under the trunk. Take an inhalation while lifting straight up the legs as high as you can. Hold the position and the breath, and then come back down exhaling. Repeat the exercise three to four times and take a rest in the initial position.

CONCENTRATION: Upon the lumbar column.

RESPIRATION: As indicated with the posture.

RESULTS: Exerts a powerful action upon the muscles of the lumbar region.

HORIZONTAL STRETCH LEGS
POSTURE (Hasta-Padangushthasana)

EXECUTION: Standing up in a relaxed position, straighten out your right leg, lift it up horizontally and catch it with the right hand. Fold the left arm behind the back. You are now standing on one leg. Try to maintain your balance and remain in the posture as long as you can. After some time, straighten the same leg out backward, and then keep it up as high as possible while remaining in the same position. And finally, bring it back to starting point. Change the position of the legs and the arms and then repeat the exercise as much as you want on each side.

CONCENTRATION: Upon the exercise.

RESPIRATION: Slow and normal. When moving the leg, do so with the rhythm of the breath.

RESULTS: It strengthens the muscles of the thighs, works upon the joints, and develops the sense of equilibrium.

HERO'S POSTURE (Virasana)

This asana is performed mostly to practice different *Bhandhas* (locks).

EXECUTION: Sit on the floor, bend the right leg and place the foot on the half part of the left thigh. Bend the left leg and cross it upon the right leg and let the left foot sit on the half part of the right thigh. You are now sitting in the half-crossed leg posture or *Padmasana*. Place both hands flat on the thighs, and bend the chin down against the jugular notch (below the throat). Exhale the air completely and hollow the stomach holding the breath. To make the bandha more accurate, bend the body forward a little and let its weight rest on the hands.

CONCENTRATION: Upon the *Manipur* chakra, situated at the navel region.

RESPIRATION: As indicated in the posture.

RESULTS: It is an excellent posture which stimulates internal abdominal massage.

THE REVERSE ADAMANTINE POSTURE (Supta Vajrasana)
FIRST POSTURE

EXECUTION: Sit down on the floor between the legs, move the bust backward with the help of the hands, and then keep the fingers interlaced on the belly. Keep on the floor the shoulder blades, the buttocks, and the front part of the feet along with the legs. The head is also resting on the nape of the neck. Hold the posture as long as you can, and then breathe normally. Finally, with the help of the hands, come back to the initial position.

CONCENTRATION: Upon the intestines.

RESPIRATION: Slow and normal.

RESULTS: This posture acts tremendously upon the digestive organs. It helps to alleviate constipation problems, affects the feet, knees, legs, joints, and the muscles.

VARIANT (Second Posture)

EXECUTION: From the same starting position of the first posture, instead of sitting between the legs, keep them close to each other and then bend yourself backward with the help of the elbows and the hands.

The whole body is now resting on the forehead; the legs and the feet are flat on the floor. The buttock is up and the hands are resting upon the thighs. Breathe normally and hold the posture as long as you can, and then with the help of the elbows and the hands, come back forward to the starting position.

CONCENTRATION: The same.

RESPIRATION: Slow and normal

RESULTS: The same as in the previous posture, but it affects the thyroid glands and strengthens the lumbar spine.

THE SCIENCE OF BREATHING (Pranayama)

KAPALABHATI PRANAYAMA

This pranayama exercise is designed to remove *Kapha* (impurities) from the respiratory tract. Its technique as described in the *Hatha Yoga Pradipika* includes rapid inhalations like the bellows of a blacksmith.

EXECUTION: Assuming a suitable posture, keep the anus and pelvis contracted. Rapid exhalations are made one after another without allowing the chest to expand or to contract appreciably. Every exhalation is brought about here mainly by sudden contraction of the abdominal muscles, causing the abdominal viscera to be pushed back by making an impact on the diaphragm, which gets raised up in the thoracic cavity, expelling some air out of the lungs through the nose. This is immediately followed by a relaxation of the abdominal muscles, causing the diaphragm to descend down in the abdominal cavity, and allowing some air to rush into the lungs through the nose as a result of this descent of the diaphragm. Afterward, another exhalation is made without losing any time. The whole process is repeated several times.

CONCENTRATION: Keep the eyes focused on the tip of the nose, and the chin is set against the jugular notch (below the throat).

THERAPEUTIC RESULTS: As traditionally believed, it makes the respiratory tract free of impurities. It renders a very valuable help in increasing one's capacity to hold the breath in or out.

BHRAMARI PRANAYAMA (The Bumble Bee)

EXECUTION: Sit in any comfortable posture. First take a deep exhalation, which is followed by an inhalation; and then exhale the air slowly through both nostrils while imitating the bee's sound in the throat center (with the chin set against the jugular notch). Take another deep inhalation and then slowly exhale the air in the same way. Repeat the cycle several times as much as you can and then take a rest.

CONCENTRATION: Focus the attention on the throat center (Vishuddha chakra) and listen to the sound which is coming out of the throat.

THERAPEUTIC RESULTS: It helps in the development of mental concentration. It purifies the throat channel from excess phlegm.

☙

LESSON 8   PART 3
HIGHER YOGA
The Technique Of Kriya Yoga

This kriya yoga we are about to teach is quite different from the commonly known Kriya Yoga, which means are to clean the internal organs by exoteric cleaning processes. Although the word *kriya* has different meanings, it really means to practice, to cure, to act, to perform purificatory rite or expiratory rite. In the kriya yoga we are about to describe, the word is used in the sense of a subtle esoteric aspect of yoga. It is also used in the sense of mudras, or symbolic gestures. The hatha yoga exercises purified and prepared the body for the understanding of kriya yoga. In hatha yoga, the movements are performed voluntarily with the power of the limbs, which are under the control of the performer. While in the esoteric kriya yoga, the movements, which are now called mudras, happen automatically. The performer is just following the movement of the prana in the body. The awakening of prana is known as *Prana Uttana*. This stage is one of the most difficult steps in yoga. It is also a stage in Hatha Yoga, where the practice becomes effortless and more enjoyable; and without it, no real divine experiences are possible.

How to awake the prana in the body?

This great blessing of the awakening of prana in the body may happen in different circumstances. The first step is the preparation of the gross physical body by a regular practice of asanas and pranayamas. Besides these, one must have a deep sincere thirst for spiritual knowledge. Someone with great artistic sensitivity is best qualified for this energy to be awakened.

Usually it could happen by a divine contact with a yogi master, and this is the best available proof for a sincere *sadhaka* to find out in his or her own body whether the guru is an authentic yogi or not. Because a master without his or her own awakened prana is not a real master.

The word *guru* means "the one who can dissipate darkness in the heart of the deserving disciple" by giving his grace in transferring a dose of his own developed prana energy into the disciple's ethereal body. From this stage of awakening, the disciple should have no more doubt concerning the guru's knowledge, because the student now should be ready to experience the yoga knowledge within his or her own body. In other words, his faith is now based in the working shakti within the body and not necessarily in the guru.

However, if the student still has doubts after the concrete manifestation of this mysterious divine (shakti) within his own body, that means that he has doubts even about the existence of his own heartbeats. This is an indication that the ego is still very strong and may be thinking that he or she has seen God, and there is no need for a guru. If he or she is unable to calm the fire of the ego, the awakening of the divine prana will soon die out without producing anything. It is similar to a seed which has been sowed on apparently prepared soil, but for some unknown reasons it does not develop or produces stunted growth.

A powerful master has the ability to awaken the prana by direct contact—by touch, by shaking hands, by thought, or just by a glance at the eyes. You can also get your prana awakened by a disciple of the master who, himself or herself, is awakened. It is just like a lighted candle can light up another candle. However, the quality and the degree of the awakening will depend on from whom it is received. If you have studied mathematics with a simple elementary school teacher, you cannot expect to get the same knowledge if you had studied with a post-graduate university professor. Your spiritual development may depend on the quality of the "pranic seed," which has been imparted in your ethereal body. After the awakening, the sadhaka needs the continuous guidance of the master in order to properly develop the shakti.

It has been said in the previous chapter that prana is the first primordial life force. So a rare master who has this life force awakened and highly developed in the body represents indeed the material manifestation of prana on earth. When a master imparts his or her own prana into someone, he has given to that person a part of his own life. So, the more the harmonious integration can be between the shakti of the disciple and the shakti of the master, the much better it is in the interest of the disciple. The wish of all authentic yogic masters is to transfer prana to as many sadhakas as possible, so that more real spiritual light can enlighten dark places in the world.

Prana can be more easily awakened in the body of young people. The younger the physical body is, the more one can feel the manifestation of prana in it. When prana is awakened, the whole body becomes spiritualized and the faith in a Supreme Being is increased in the heart of the sadhaka.

MANIFESTATION OF PRANA

For esoteric reasons, we are not able to give all the details of the manifestation of prana in the body. We will only give the essential in order to draw your attention to it. After all, it is a personal experience which will be useful only to the one who is experiencing it.

Usually to perform the hatha yoga exercises you need the help of your will. Sometimes the will is not strong enough to help you to follow regularly the discipline, to get up early in the morning, and to start with the practice. In kriya yoga, since the movements are performed automatically, you do not need the help of the ordinary will anymore. The divine will of the guru inside of your own self will perform the asanas for you.

During the practice, whatever is hidden in your subconscious will come out. Your artistic talents will be revealed to you. You will sing, dance, laugh, and weep. According to your own compassionate tendency, you might feel universal love in your heart (the love of Christ). You will understand the meaning of all religions. You will become self-confident. The more you remain humble in your heart with full respect for the mysterious awakening shakti in your body, the more you will progress spiritually.

The practice of yoga will be a greater pleasure to you. After practicing it regularly, willfully, you will then let prana do the subtle work for you. This is the best way to purify the physical and the ethereal body.

If the grace of the master is always upon you, by your sincerity and your good deeds you will be able to get access to higher stages of yoga. One obstacle to keep in mind in kriya yoga is the EGO. Sometimes after a few months or a couple of years of practice, a sadhaka with a strong ego may feel that he or she does not need the guru anymore, and starts behaving as his or her own guru. The result is that such sadhaka will never be able to get access to higher stages of *Raja Yoga*, and sooner or later she will move in different directions. In all the yoga Upanishad, the *rishis* have always warned the sadhakas about the danger of the ego. We found similar warning in the teaching of Jesus Christ, when he said to his disciples, "If you don't remain as a child, you shall never get access to the kingdom of my Father."

The Prana Uttana stage is very difficult to obtain for the one who is not fit for it. It is also the first necessary stage in higher yoga. Without it, there is no real yoga, which leads to the road of self-realization.

However, for the selfish and the self-centered sadhaka who has not overcome the ego problem, persisting in the adventure of esoteric kriya yoga could lead to madness. We have heard of students reporting uncontrollable visual and auditory hallucinations leading to anxiety and mental disturbances. Kriya yoga practice should not lead to the symptoms of schizophrenia, unless the student has an evil motive to misuse the knowledge.

In India, out of one thousand monks (sanyasi), it is very difficult to find one who really has knowledge of kriya yoga or who has the prana awakened in the body. This knowledge is transmitted from guru to disciple. And if you have a guru who is not awakened, then how can you expect to get awakened? Light can only come from a light source and not from darkness. For further details, if you feel that you have a desire to be enlightened, then you should seek an enlightened master who will guide you on this path.

CHAPTER XI

THE POSTURES (ASANAS)

I n this lesson we will start with the study of some more advanced asanas. We cannot tell in advance which student can easily succeed in such or such asana. This depends upon the morphological constitution of each student's body, on the practice, and on the natural flexibility of the limbs. Sometimes a student may easily succeed in mastering a difficult asana and fail in a very simple one. Let us specify that there are three stages in the mastering of a posture:

1-You have to learn how to perform it well.

2-You have to be able to hold it a certain period of time.

3-You have to be completely relaxed while maintaining the posture.

THE FOOT-TIED TREE POSTURE
(Ardha-Baddhapadma-Vrikshasana)

EXECUTION: This posture is performed from the second tree posture. Standing up, bend the left leg, catch it up with the hands and place it upon the right thigh with the sole facing upward. Turn the left arm behind the hip and catch the toes of the left foot. Try to maintain your balance and do not bend forward. Hold the posture as long as possible then bring the leg down and reverse the position.

CONCENTRATION: Upon the mental and physical balance.

BREATHING: Slow and regular.

RESULTS: Makes a powerful work upon the knee articulations and develops the sense of balance.

VARIANT OF THE HORIZONTAL-STRETCH LEG
POSTURE (Hasta-Padangushthasana)

EXECUTION: This is performed in the same way as the horizontal leg posture. The only difference is that the hands are catching the toes of the opposite foot.

Standing up, fold the left leg and catch the toes with the right hand. Keep the leg and the arm as straight as possible in the horizontal position. Place the left hand behind the back at the lumbar region. Hold the posture as long as possible without shaking. After some time, change the leg and reverse the position.

CONCENTRATION: Upon the physical and the mental balance.

BREATHING: Slow and regular

RESULTS: It brings suppleness to the hips, the posterior thigh muscles, and increases the sense of physical and mental balance.

THE LION POSTURE (Simhasana)

EXECUTION: Sit down on the heels, cross the ankles upon each other. The knees are resting on the floor. Keep the hands clenched on the knees with straight arms. Take a deep breath through both nostrils. Exhale the air through the mouth while pulling the tongue out as much as possible. Increase the movement by pressing the fists upon the knees, and keep the chin down. The bust is erect, and keep the tongue out a few seconds. Repeat this exercise three to four times. Slowly give up the position and relax the legs.

CONCENTRATION: Upon the throat center.

BREATHING: Just as described with the posture.

RESULTS: It exerts a powerful action upon the throat and the tonsils which are washed by the rush of the blood.

THIRD VARIANT OF THE JANUSHIR POSTURE
(Janushirasana)

EXECUTION: Sit with straight legs, bend the right leg and place the sole of the foot near the left thigh. You are in the student posture. Now bend slowly towards the straight leg and then catch your left leg with the left hand; the elbow is touching the floor. Pass the right arm upon the head and catch the toes of the left leg with the right hand. Hold the posture as long as possible. After some time, slowly give it up and reverse the position.

CONCENTRATION: Upon the spinal column.

BREATHING: Slow and regular.

RESULTS: It brings suppleness to the posterior thigh muscles and affects the trunk muscles and the knee's articulations. It also exerts a powerful action upon the internal abdominal organs, the pancreas, and the adrenal glands.

THE WATCHER POSTURE (Prekshasana)

EXECUTION: Lie down on the belly, and place the hands near the shoulders. The feet are straight and close to each other. Slowly rise up the body; the arms are straight, and take only the support of the fingers and the toes. Repeat the exercise 4 to 6 times, and every time you raise up the body, maintain the position a few seconds.

CONCENTRATION: Upon the vertebral axis.

BREATHING: Rhythmically.

RESULTS: This exercise acts upon the toes, the fingers, and the pectoral muscles. It also helps to develop control over the physical body.

THE SOLITARY FOOT POSTURE (Ekapadashirasana)

EXECUTION: Sit on the floor with both legs straight. Bend the left leg and catch the left ankle with both hands. The left arm is off the left knee. Push backwards the leg and the left thigh until the underknee comes to sit upon the left shoulder. The left leg is then parallel to the floor. The right leg is resting straight on the floor. Keep the hands folded together behind the back. The pressure of the left arm on the back permits to maintain a horizontal position of the left leg. Hold the posture as long as you can, and then change the leg and reverse the position.

CONCENTRATION: Upon the posture.

BREATHING: Slow and regular.

RESULTS: It brings suppleness to the hips, the joints, and strength to the shoulder muscles.

THE BIRD POSTURE (Khagasana)

EXECUTION: Lying flat on the belly, bend the legs and catch the toes. Work them up by pressing them gently and try to bring the heels near the buttocks. At the same time, raise the head and the bust up as high as possible. The knees are separated from each other, and the elbows are in an upright position. Hold the posture as long as possible and then take a rest on the starting position.

CONCENTRATION: Slow and regular.

RESULTS: It increases the flexibility of the knees and the ankle joints. It may prevent rheumatism in the joints; it also strengthens the thyroid gland and the back muscles.

THE SCIENCE OF BREATHING (Pranayama)

The pranayama which we are about to describe is one of the most important pranayama in yogic literature. In the beginning, it must be performed carefully and should not be done excessively.

THE BELLOWS PRANAYAMA (Bastrika)

This pranayama is performed in a noisy way; that is why it is called the blowing pranayama. While performing this pranayama you should feel an increased current of prana entering the ethereal body, which may produce a little sensation of dizziness. This will show to you the efficacy of the pranayama. After performing it a few times, take rest in shavasana.

EXECUTION: Sit in any comfortable posture and keep the spine erect, and take a deep inhalation and exhalation according to the procedure of complete breathing. The difference is in the rhythm, which is short and fast. You should not bother with the counting time of inhalation and exhalation.

Repeat the exercise ten times, meaning: ten times of inhalation and exhalation. At the eleventh time, take a deep inhalation, hold the breath a few seconds, and then exhale slowly. You may as you wish perform the cycle three to four times.

CONCENTRATION: Upon the breathing rhythm.

RESULTS: It raises the current of prana up in the body. It heats up the body and cleans up the respiratory system.

LESSON 9   **PART 2**

HIGHER YOGA
The Possible Obstacles in Meditation
and How to Avoid Them

Many obstacles may come in the way of the student who has started practicing meditation without discrimination. Before starting seriously the practice of meditation, one must get proper guidance from a qualified guru and the rules of Yama-Niyama should be put to application.

However, the student who practices ordinary meditation for no more than half an hour a day has nothing to fear about, because in that beginning stage the vibrations generated by the mind are not powerful enough to bring any transcendental experiences.

The obstacles may come in the way of a beginner sadhaka who is practicing long hours of meditation with powerful mental concentration, without proper guidance and knowledge.

We do not advise to the student who is not able yet to meet a guru to practice any kind of meditation alone in a room. If he or she wishes to do so, it must be collective, where the vibration currents are concentrating in one ethereal body.

During the practice of deep meditation some powerful energy currents are liberated from the cosmic field and invade the psychic centers (the chakras) of the sadhaka. The chakras transmit the energies to the nervous system, the endocrine glands, and the nervous cells of the body. The nervous system, the glands, and the whole body complex must be able to adjust themselves and to withstand the invasion of such powerful energies. The adjustment of the body can only be slowed progressively. The regular practice of hatha yoga and a moderate way of living should prepare the body and the mind to face such stages in meditation. It is important for the student in the initial stage to carefully watch the psycho-physiological reactions in meditation.

THE MENTAL REACTION – To approach the superior region where the contact is possible with the higher spirit, the sadhaka must quiet the waves of the lower mentality. To pacify the mental is one of the most important steps in the process of meditation. How to obtain it?

One can succeed only by regular proper exercises performed careful-ly. A violent intervention of the willpower is not desirable. It can only produce an inhibition which will have a direct effect upon the physical brain and will lead to fatigue or drowsiness.

After meditation, one should not feel tired. If it happens, it means that you are putting up much stress somewhere. You must always watch your physical state after meditation. However, in the beginning, since the nerves and the muscles have not yet cleaned, a little discomfort after meditation is quite normal and should not worry you.

Try to learn how to pacify the mental thoughts by some exercises which should be performed at the same hour in a quiet place. During that time, you must keep the physical body relaxed, breathe slowly, and control the emotional body. You should not forget that the mental should not dominate the emotional and the physical bodies in such a way to annihilate them. The truth is in the right adjustment of the three lower bodies—physical, mental, emotional—which should become a divine instrument at the disposal of the soul and permit it to rise up at different manifested levels.

THE EMOTIONAL REACTIONS – The common human of our time is polarized in the astral or emotional body, also called sensual body. The control of this body is especially difficult to obtain. In most people, the sensual body has become one with the physical, and the physical automatically obeys its injunctions. The real yogi is the one who has detached the physical body from the sensual and who has placed the sensual body directly under the control of the divine kundalini shakti.

THE PHYSICAL REACTIONS – We have said that the practice of meditation attracts a great amount of cosmic energy in the chakras, and consequently liberates some high currents of magnetic energies in the physical body.

Another physical and mental reaction which may come to the selfish sadhaka who is trying to awake the chakras by some special exaggerated yogic breathing in order to gain some physical power (*siddhis*) is madness. However, for the sincere sadhaka who is practicing meditation only for spiritual advancement there is no danger, and on the way he or she shall be blessed by an auspicious meeting with the guru, who will provide guidance.

In addition, the student who is practicing meditation without observing the rules, instead of gaining calmness may feel agitated, impatient, and nervous. Such student should then give up the meditation and practice karma yoga and hatha yoga to purify the body and the mind.

Note about kundalini shakti: This is our first allusion in this book about it. We have tried to avoid this subject which can be taught only and directly to a fit sadhaka by a realized yogi guru.

CHAPTER XII

NATURAL LIFE
The Secret of Health and Longevity

The yogis prefer to live in places where the nature is green, where there are plenty of trees, fresh air, and clean water. In such places, they are in permanent communication with nature and cosmic vibrations. They are fully aware of the life which is in everything; that is why they don't kill anything, and they respect life in all of its different forms. They like to expose the body to the air, to the salutary sun rays, to fresh water of the rivers and the sea. They prefer to practice yoga and meditation in deep wooded areas, where the purest oxygen is available and to better attract cosmic energies.

Natural forest and floras have a beneficial influence upon the health. They constitute an inexhaustible reservoir of peace and vitality. Every time you have the opportunity to get away from cities and crowded places, take advantage of the moment to go away and recharge the body and the mind. You will find in the open country a faithful friend.

Some places are more beneficial for the human health than others, such as hill stations, seaside resorts, and pine forests. If you have the chance to be in those places, take any opportunity to practice pranayama. On the seashore, you have freely at your disposal one of the four natural elements known by ancient sages and which they used in their natural therapeutic cure, which is the sand heated by the sun, which they believe has the ability to relieve rheumatism. Seawater is the best therapy to regenerate the body. Salubrious air charged with ozone and iodide vivifies the organisms. The sun brings vitality in the form of prana to the body cells.

You should often use the free gift of nature. However, the sun should be used carefully, because it is well-known that too much exposure to sun rays could be harmful to health. Indeed, one should take a deep bath in nature and love her sincerely. She also, as the poet said, loves you and is inviting you. She is offering to you her changing symphony at the rhythm of the seasons. Try to penetrate the mysteries with a heart full of love. One day, your soul will mix its note with the cosmic song.

HEALTH AND LONG LIFE

The problem of longevity has always puzzled humanity. During all the previous centuries, medical doctors, alchemists, and magicians have searched for the supreme secret which was supposed to prolong life. Mixtures of powders, salt, secret elixirs of long life, and youthful water have been put at the disposal of credulous people, without any significant results. Now-a-days modern science is still searching for the magic pill which they think will prolong life way beyond the normal life expectancy. We are often bombarded with advertised new discoveries of promising health care products, of youthful body and a long life.

If the average of human life has gone up, mostly in developed countries, it is basically due to better health care. However, we do not count anymore those who are struck down between forty and fifty years of age. Although the number of centenarians has increased, the quality of life of those folks is not much desirable.

Indeed, the possibility of living a long healthy life beyond 100 is real. In Western countries as well as in Asian countries we found in old scriptures some extraordinary cases of longevity (Babylonians, Greeks, Romans, Indians, and Chinese). In the Bible, we found quite a great number of patriarchs who are believed to have lived between 700 to 900 years (Genesis 3:15). If we have doubt about them, we cannot ignore the case of Moses, an historical personage who was reported to have lived 120 years; and which at that age was able to climb Mount Nebo (Genesis 33.2). Even today, deep in the Balkan, in the Caucasian countries, and in the high Tibetan Himalayan region, people aged close to Moses or beyond have been reported (Collison, D. 2006). It is well-documented about the lifespan of 140 years or more of the Hunza, a tribe living deep in the Himalayas. We could state that the human body has been created to live at least one century, upon the condition of maintaining it well.

Through the regular holistic yoga practice, you have the opportunity to maintain the youthfulness of the organs of the body. By its influence upon all the great organic functions and mostly upon the nervous system and the endocrine gland, yoga can help to maintain in perfect condition the human body and extend the quality of life. The wear-out of different organs can be delayed to the maximum, and the diseases can be defeated by the vitality of the physiological organs.

It is evident that if the beats of the heart are slowed down, the heart will last longer. If the food diet is pure and well balanced, the blood vessels will undergo fewer alterations. If the nervous system is calmed and stress free, the sadakha will master old age. If the spinal column remains flexible, the life energy will spread throughout better. If the respiration is complete, the blood oxygenation will always be optimum, and the cells of the body will be renewed properly.

According to the yogis, the secret of long life is hidden in the way a person breathes. Breathing brings life and if it stops, death will come. When a person comes into this world, teach the yogis, he or she has a certain number of breaths to effectuate. If one breathes too fast, the life will be shortened. On the contrary, if one learns to control the breath, the length of life will be extended. In this chapter, you have been given the secret of long life, and for your own benefit try to experiment it within yourself.

ॐ

LESSON 10   **PART 2**
THE ASANAS

THE STORK POSTURE (Vakasana)
To perform this posture requires quite a great suppleness of the lumbar spine and the posterior thigh muscles, which by now you should have.

EXECUTION: Stand up, with feet close to each other, and keep the arms alongside the body. Take a deep inhalation; slowly bend the bust forwards, while exhaling until the forehead touches the knees if possible. Catch the ankles of both feet and hold the position as long as possible. While holding the posture, breathe normally in order to remain in it for a longer time. Afterward, inhale and come back up to the starting position and breathe normally. Repeat the exercise 3 to 4 times.

CONCENTRATION: Upon the lumbar region.

RESPIRATION: As indicated in the posture.

RESULTS: It makes the lumbar column more flexible and strengthens the posterior muscles of the thighs. It also exerts a powerful action upon the abdominal organs and the endocrine glands, and irrigates the brain with fresh blood.

GOKARNASANA (The Cow's Ear Posture)

EXECUTION: Lying on the back with straight legs, the arms alongside the body, bend the right leg, catch the toes of the right foot with the right hand and slowly stretch the right leg, and the right arm, until they become straight flat on the floor. Now the right leg is supposed to be perpendicular with the left one, and form about a 90-degree angle with the left leg. Keep the left arm straight and flat on the floor in the same line with the left leg. Hold the posture as long as you can and try to keep your back flat on the floor. After a while, give up the posture and reverse the position.

CONCENTRATION: Upon the posture.

RESPIRATION: Slow and regular.

RESULTS: This posture reinforces the suppleness of the posterior muscles of the thighs and the lateral muscles of the trunks.

REALIZATION POSTURE (Muktasana)

This posture has two variants.

POSTURE 1

EXECUTION: Sit on the left heel with the leg bent under the buttocks, catch the right foot and place it upon the left thigh. The sole of the foot is facing upwards and both knees are flat on the floor. Keep the bust erect and the hands resting on the knees. Remain in the position as long as possible. After a while, reverse the position of the legs.

CONCENTRATION: Upon the *Anahat chakra* (at the heart region).

RESPIRATION: Normal and regular.

RESULTS: This is a physical and psychical balance posture. It regularizes the nervous current in the body, which is favorable for the practice of mediation and pranayama.

POSTURE 2

EXECUTION: From the first posture we have described as follows: The left heel is under the buttocks and right foot is resting upon the left thigh. Catch behind the back the wrist of one hand with the other. Inhale deeply and slowly, bend the bust forwards in exhaling. Touch the floor with the forehead if possible and hold on the breath. Then after a few seconds, come up with an inhalation and breathe normally. Repeat this exercise three times on each side.

CONCENTRATION: Upon the *Ajna Chakra* (between the eyebrows).

RESPIRATION: As indicated with posture.

RESULTS: It improves the flexibility of the lumbar spine, the joints of the ankles, and the knees. It also affects the abdominal organs and activates the current of prana in the Ajna chakra.

LIFT UP POSTERIOR STRENGTH POSTURE
(Utthita-Sarvangasana)

EXECUTION: Sit on the floor with bent legs close to each other. Catch the big toes with two fingers of each hand. Stretch straight the legs, the arms, and remain sitting only on the buttocks. The forehead should be close to the knees. Try to keep your balance and hold the posture as long as you can. Repeat the exercise 3 to 4 times and then take a rest in Shavasana position.

CONCENTRATION: Upon the balance in the posture.

RESPIRATION: Regular.

RESULTS: This posture works powerfully upon the abdominal lateral muscles of the trunk and the lumbar column. The abdominal cavity organs, along with the endocrinal glands are regenerated. The sense of physical and psychical balance is increased.

VARIANT OF THE HALF POSTURE OF MATSYENDRA
(Ardha-Matsyendrasana)

EXECUTION: Sit on the floor, with the left leg bent and the heel near the buttocks. Bend the right leg and cross it upon the left thigh. The right foot is now flat on the floor near the left knee. Turn over the right arm behind the back and catch if possible the right foot with the right hand. Pass the straight left arm over in the front of the right knee and catch the left knee with the left hand. Hold the posture as long as possible and then reverse the position. Repeat the exercise three times on each side.

CONCENTRATION: Upon the spinal column.

RESPIRATION: Slow and regular.

RESULTS: This posture may rectify scoliosis; it acts upon the ganglions of the sympathetic system. It acts upon the liver, the pancreas, and the intestines.

THE TURTLE POSTURE (Kurmasana)

EXECUTION: Sit on the floor. The legs and the thighs are separated as much as possible. Bend forward the head and the bust. Squeeze the arms under the thighs and straighten them up behind. By pressing the arms and the hands hard on the floor, the forward flexion is increased, and the head gets nearer to the ground. Hold the posture as long as you can while breathing slowly. After a while, give up the posture and take rest. Repeat the exercise 3 to 4 times.

CONCENTRATION: Upon the thyroid gland (the throat center).

RESPIRATION: Slow and superficial.

RESULTS: It provides flexibility to the spinal column, mostly at the lumbar region. It also strengthens the sympathetic ganglions, massages the thyroid gland, reinvigorates the nervous system, and increases the digestive function.

CAMEL POSTURE (Ushtrasana)

This posture looks like the bow posture we already have studied; however, it is somewhat more difficult.

EXECUTION: Lying flat on the belly, bend the legs upon each other; the feet are crossed upon the buttocks. Cross the arms behind the back and catch the feet. The right arm is catching the left foot, and the left arm is catching the right foot. Take a deep inhalation and raise the head and the bust up, while stretching upon the feet. The knees are above the ground. Stay in the posture and hold the breath as long as possible with empty lungs. After some time, release the tension, come down and exhale without giving up the position.

CONCENTRATION: Upon the posture.

RESPIRATION: As described in the posture

RESULTS: It strengthens the spinal, the back, and the trapeze muscles. It stimulates the endocrine gland, the pancreas, and the sexual glands. It also acts upon the liver and kidneys, and it corrects certain defects of the ovaries.

THE SCIENCE OF BREATHING (Pranayama)

The pranayama series which will be taught in this lesson and in the 11th and the 12th lessons are useful to purify the nadis before the practice of meditation. However, the students who are not interested in meditation may leave them aside and practice only those previously taught. Their practices may produce some powerful spiritual and psychological effects which could really be beneficial to a student, but only if one follows the rules of higher yoga.

THE TRIANGLE BREATHING (Tribhuja Pranayama)

EXECUTION: This pranayama is performed with the rhythm of 12-12-12. Sit in any comfortable posture, inhale for 12 seconds, and hold the breath 12 seconds, while concentrating upon the *Ajna chakra*. Exhale completely for 12 seconds and breathe normally. Repeat this exercise as many times as you want, without exaggerating.

CONCENTRATION: Upon the Ajna Chakra (between the eyebrows).

REMARKS: The inhalation must be very slow in order to last for the 12 seconds. From the beginning of the inhalation, you should take all the care to protect yourself, and the rest will automatically follow.

THE SATURATED BREATHING (Atisikta Pranayama)

EXECUTION: Sit in any comfortable posture, take a deep inhalation, but in a particular jerking way. Jerk the air regularly, but slowly, slowly, until the lungs become full of air. This inhalation is constituted of a succession of small inhalations, each separate with a short retention.

When the lungs are filled up with the air, hold the breath according to your own capacity, between 12-16- or 24 seconds. Then exhale through both nostrils as slowly as possible.

CONCENTRATION: During the retention upon the Ajna Chakra.

ॐ

LESSON 10   **PART 3**

HIGHER YOGA

The Importance of Breathing in the Spiritual Transformation

(Life and Yogic Breathing)

We already have said that perfect health is the basic condition to succeed with the practice of meditation and to advance further on the spiritual path. Controlled breathing, which leads to the rectification of the physiological and vital functions, is indispensable for the sadhaka in order to maintain a body fit for higher experiences.

In this short chapter, we will explore a little further the physiological effects of controlled breathing. We will examine the basic pranayamas which you will be using most of the time. Let us see what those pranayamas are:

The complete and deep breathing – The rhythmic breathing – The alternate breathing – The pranayama with breath retention.

Our first verification is this: Normal, ordinary breathing brings a reduced pulmonary ventilation, while the pranayamas we have quoted increased considerably the volume of inhaled and exhaled air.

Normal inhalation brings about .5 liter of air into the lungs, while deep complete inhalation will bring about a maximum of 2 liters, which means much more than the normal inhalation. In the same way, the total exhalation expels a great quantity of air in comparison with normal exhalation.

By the practice of pranayama, considerable pulmonary ventilation arises in the body, which brings about some beneficial effects to the entire body. The influx of air in the lungs produces an afflux of oxygen (the vital gas), which carries life to the body cells.

It is through the blood hemoglobin that the gaseous circuit of the respiration is formed, in which the outside oxygen comes to modify the internal composition of the body and permits life to develop. In the same manner, the internal gaseous wastes are discharged outside to permit a new coming of fresh material energies.

The whole process is performed in a rhythm comparable with the flux and the reflux of the ocean and the great cosmic rhythms. The complete yogic breathing acts directly upon the blood circulation by the modification of the intra-thoracic and intra-abdominal pressures. The inhalation provokes a diminution of pressure in the thoracic cage and increases the pressure in the abdominal cavity, while the exhalation does the contrary. Some sanguine currents are produced in opposite direction of those influences, which as a result activate the blood circulation in the body.

The deep yogic breathing also has an influence upon nutrition. It regularizes the degree of gastric acidity and intestinal alkaline. It also allows the normal combustion of the hydrate carbonic, the greases and their right utilization in the organism. Some vitamins are in need of plenty oxygen to be properly utilized in the body. For this the yogic pranayamas may serve the purpose.

The endocrine glands, mostly the thyroid, are regenerated by a great afflux of oxygen. The thyroid gland which regularizes the basic metabolism of the body can be readjusted by the regular practice of complete yogic breathing. This breathing influences also the adrenal gland and the production of sex hormones (Schaeffer, M.R. et al., 2014).

This short discourse, which is inserted in the frame of actual medical knowledge, shows you how various pranayamas transmitted to us by the ancient yogi masters are favorable for the maintenance of health, a basic condition for the discovery of the self.

BREATH AND THE HOLY SPIRIT

The existing homology between the breath and the Holy Spirit constitutes the great discovery of the ancient sages. In all the great esoteric doctrines, the importance of breath has been underscored. According to the tradition, it is while meditating upon the breath that the Buddha Gautama was enlightened. It is for this reason that we will now study the spiritual effects of pranayama, after going through its psycho-chemical and physiological effects.

On a lower plane, pranayama influences and modifies life of the body. In the same way it will also modify, on a superior level, the subtle vehicles of the body. There is a close relationship between the breath and various psychic techniques which modify the length of the breath. Consequently, during meditation such techniques provoke a transformation of different conscious states. Just as life is the manifestation of different conscious states, it is the whole life of a being which is transformed by the effect of pranayama.

Let us examine the three successive phases of conscious breathing in humans. First of all, we inhale and exhale the planetary air, and fill up the lungs and the whole being with the prana. We then receive divine life on all levels.

In a second phase, we retain the breath and concentrate on the inside of the self, the divine force or the divine prana. It is the balance period between the two phases—inhalation and exhalation. During this retention, we are in full balance with our whole being, realizing the contact with the soul and receiving the subtle energies from the true inner self. This synergy is the result of powerful concentration and deep meditation, which gives access to the superior world of above. At last, in a third phase, the adept, by the process of exhalation, has freed the self from the tension of accumulating forces and restored them back to the cosmic field.

MENTAL CONCENTRATION UPON THE BREATH

The mental concentration is a simple method to settle the mind and permits the adept to go further towards different superior stages of concentration, meditation, and visualization. In those comfortable postures such as Sukhasana Padmasana, the adept is preparing by corporal stillness for this deep concentration.

The adept performs various pranayamas while trying to isolate the time length of inhalation, retention, and exhalation. He or she carefully counts the different periods while chasing out all negative thoughts in the mind. At the same time, she must visualize and create the image in the mind while breathing in the air through the nostrils. She also follows the pulmonary rhythm, the extension and compression of the lungs, and the diaphragm movements which rhythmically lower and raise them up. The adept's entire consciousness identifies itself mentally and biologically with the respiratory action.

At the end, the adept visualizes the afflux of prana with the breath. She also sees moving in the nadis the subtle energy which is spreading and vitalizing the chakras of the ethereal body, accumulating in this way divine forces in the body.

By the regular practice of those techniques, the adept is preparing to accede to higher different stages, but at the same time she vitalizes her ethereal body and pacifies the mental, where calmness, joy, and peace come to dwell permanently.

THE COSMIC BREATHING

This breathing is also a step in superior initiation and cannot be entirely revealed. On the human point of view, it can be compared with the great vital air which animates the universe.

There are four tempos in it: inhalation, breath retention (with full lungs), exhalation, and breath retention (with empty lungs). There is also a similar breathing with retention, which we will study in the 12th lesson. The difference in the cosmic breathing is justified by the activity performed during the two tempos of retention. It is supplemented with deep meditation and a higher soul is added to the simple starting movements of prana.

In superior retention the adept is conscious of the divine energies which are flowing in the body. In the lower retention (with empty lungs), she restores those energies on a material level and participates in this way in the process of the evolution.

CHAPTER XIII

LESSON 11   **PART 1**

THE ACTION OF YOGA UPON THE SPINAL COLUMN

The one who practices regularly the psycho-physiological science of yoga we have described shall become his or her own physician. The asanas, the pranayama, mental concentration, and meditation have powerful progressive influence upon the human organism, which they maintain or restore to health.

In this lesson we will examine the mechanical effects of the asanas upon the spinal column. Of course, yoga is one whole technique; the pranayamas and concentration will not be forgotten and should work together with the asanas.

The spinal column plays an essential role in the human complex. It constitutes the frame of the body which sustains the head and the thoracic cage. It supports the gravity action, which has a tendency to push the body on the ground. It contains and protects the spinal marrow. From the conjugation holes formed by the vertebra go out the nerves which carry the vital magnetic influx to the organs.

From this we do not have to specify any more on how the state of the spinal column has an influence upon the health of the body. None has to be a qualified osteopath to maintain this fact. We just have to take a look at a sketch of the rachis to be immediately convinced. Throughout the vertebral axis come out the nervous commands, which form the sympathetic system. Both chains of the ganglions constituting of the brachial nerves are situated on both sides of the vertebra close to them. It is obvious that any vertebral deterioration has a repercussion upon the nerves, and consequently upon the ortho-sympathetic nervous system itself. That is why osteopathy, a system of medicine, states a theory that disturbances in the musculoskeletal affect other body parts, and may be at the root of many disorders that can be corrected by various hand manipulation techniques (Gevits, N. 2004).

Maintaining the spinal column in good physiological state is one of the essential conditions of excellent health. Compared to other techniques or invasive therapy, yoga is a natural intervention that best serves the purpose. As we age, the intervertebral disc begins to lose its suppleness. It becomes harder and thinner. The ligaments slowly are worn out; the spinal muscles lose their elasticity. Mostly among sedentary people, the spinal column has a tendency to squeeze, which may accentuate the natural curvature. With the regular practice of yoga, such a process is much retarded. Most of the asanas act upon the spinal column and help to maintain or give it back its elasticity.

The slow movements performed in the asanas provoke a tremendous work out of the discs, which brings elasticity and vitality. The stretch in the postures makes the ligaments and the muscular tendons supple. The nerves which come out of the conjugation holes are strengthened and straightened out. The arteries, the veins, and the capillaries which nourish the vertebral complex are maintained in a good physical state. Blood circulation improves and may keep the spinal vertebral articulations warmer. The bones are themselves nourished with fresh blood and remain strong and alive.

With the regular practice of the asanas, the spinal column will maintain its elasticity even in old age, as can be seen in bodies of aged Indian yogis in India. Yoga also has a curative effect, as it has been reported by many yoga practitioners. Finally, we can say that the science of yoga has shown that daily practice of holistic yoga with proper diet may retard considerably the aging process in certain people.

≈

LESSON 11   **PART 2**
THE ASANAS
We are proceeding in this lesson with some more advanced postures. Usually to perform them easily requires quite a long practice. Therefore, you should not be in a hurry to take on a difficult posture if you believe that your limbs are not ready. It is essential that you proceed carefully and with insight, in order to avoid damaging any ligament.

THE HALF LEG POSTURE (Ardha-Padasana)
EXECUTION: Kneeling on the right leg bent, catch the left foot and place it tightly upon the right thigh. Help yourself with the right hand

fingers straight to the floor, searching for your balance. The left knee is on the floor, and the whole body is supported by the knees and the bent foot on the floor. Continue to search for your balance, and try to keep the spine as straight as possible. Place both hands folded at the chest level (in the form of prayer) and remain in the position as long as possible. Breathe normally, and after some time, reverse the position of the legs.

CONCENTRATION: Upon your balance in the posture.

RESPIRATION: Just follow your breathing while maintaining your equilibrium.

RESULTS: It helps in the development to the maximum of the elasticity of the knees, ankles, and increases the sense of physical and mental equilibrium.

ON THE TOES POSTURES

FIRST POSTURE

EXECUTION: Kneeling on the tip of the toes, stretch straight the right leg forward with both hands parallel on the floor. Try to maintain the balance while sitting on the tip of the toes, and keep the posture as long as you can. After some time, reverse the position.

CONCENTRATION: Upon your equilibrium in the posture.

RESPIRATION: Just follow your breathing.

RESULTS: This is a beneficial asana for mental and physical balance.

SECOND POSTURE

EXECUTION: Kneeling on the tip of the toes, catch the left foot and place it upon the right knee. You are now sitting on the toes of the right foot. Search for your balance and try to remain unshaken, and as soon as you can, place both hands folded at the chest level. After some time, reverse the position. Repeat the exercise three times on each leg.

CONCENTRATION: Upon the posture.

RESPIRATION: Slow and regular.

RESULTS: Same as in the first posture.

THE LOTUS POSTURE (Padmasana)

If you have practiced regularly the previous leg postures, you have a better chance to succeed right away in this one. However, you should not force the limbs if the joints are still stiff. Usually this asana is quite a challenge for Westerners who are not used to sit on the floor or to cross their legs. However, with some patience and perseverance, one day you should be able to perform it easily.

EXECUTION: Sit on the ground, fold the right leg and place the right foot upon the left thigh with the help of both hands. Next, fold carefully the left leg, cross it upon the other, with the foot resting upon the right thigh. Keep the spine vertical and the bust erect. Let both hands rest upon the knees, and then relax the whole body. Remain in the position as long as you can, and then reverse the position, and afterward stretch out the legs and take a rest in *Shavasana.*

CONCENTRATION: Upon the Anahat chakra, near the heart center.

RESPIRATION: Just follow the breathing.

Note: *All the pranayamas exercises can be practiced in this posture.*

RESULTS: This is the key posture of the yogis for the practice of meditation. It gives stability to the body and balances the mind. It is a good tonic for the nerves of the legs and the thighs. It also calms down the nervous system and it provides relief to rheumatism of the inferior limbs. From this posture, we will study many other asanas.

THE LION POSTURE IN LOTUS (Padmasinhasana)

EXECUTION: From the lotus posture, place the hands on the floor with straight arms. With the help of the hands, stand up on the knees and bend forwards. Open the mouth and stick out the tongue. Inhale through the nostrils, and exhale through the mouth rhythmically. Hold the posture and after some time, come back to sitting in the initial position.

CONCENTRATION: Upon the throat center (Vishuddha Chakra)

RESPIRATION: Rhythmic and slow.

RESULTS: It makes supple the articulations of the knees and the ankles. It also acts upon the throat and the tonsil to clean up and vitalize them.

GREAT PRAYER POSTURE IN LOTUS (Bhunamana Padmasana)
Note: *This asana is also a Mudra (or symbolic gesture).*
EXECUTION: From the Padmasana or crossed legs posture, place both hands behind the back and catch the left wrist with the right hand and take a deep breath; then slowly bend the bust forwards while exhaling until the forehead touches the floor. Hold the posture with empty lungs for about 12 seconds, without lifting the buttock up. Come back up slowly while inhaling, and then exhale.
CONCENTRATION: Focus the mind between the Ajna chakra at the middle of the eyebrows.
RESPIRATION: 1- As indicated with the posture; 2- If you want to hold the posture a certain length of time, just breathe slowly and regularly. In this case, do not keep the posture beyond 3 minutes.
RESULTS: This asana has a powerful psychic effect. It also acts upon the interior limbs and the lumbar spinal.

FISH POSTURE (Matsyasana)
EXECUTION: From the lotus posture in Padmasana, first place one elbow on the floor and then the other one, and then with the help of the hands, stretch completely backward. When the shoulders reach the floor, enlace the hands and cross the arms behind the head. After some time, you can also release the enlaced hand behind the neck and enlace them on the stomach. The back is now lying flat on the floor. Hold the posture as long as you can and breathe normally. Finally, to give up the asana, take a deep inhalation and come straight up and forward with the help of the hands, and then breathe normally.
CONCENTRATION: Upon the stomach.
RESPIRATION: As indicated in the posture
RESULTS: This is an excellent posture to develop the digestive power. It also increases the knees and the leg resistance. It brings supple-

ness to the hip articulations, develops the breast, the back; finally, it acts to fortify the muscles and the nerves of the neck.

THE SCIENCE OF NOSTRIL BREATHING (Pranayama)

Those two breathing types of pranayama which we are about to teach are very important for the practice of meditation and they must be performed carefully.

EXECUTION: Take a complete inhalation through the right nostril. Bend the head forwards with the chin touching the upper chest, and then hold the breath as long as possible. Exhale slowly through the right nostril and keep the head down. Take a new inhalation and raise up the head, exhale, and breathe normally through both nostrils.

CONCENTRATION: Upon the pranayama.

RESULTS: It helps in the prevention of cold in the head, gives some beneficial mental and psychological results.

EAR PRANAYAMA

EXECUTION: Close both ears with the thumbs and take a deep quick inhalation. Hold the breath with full lungs as long as you can and then exhale quickly.

CONCENTRATION: Upon the humming sound in the ears.

RESULTS: Better pranic circulation in the entire nervous system, leading to mental clarity and psychological wellbeing.

ॐ

LESSON 11   PART 3

HIGHER YOGA
The Yoga of The New Age
(Karma Yoga, or Selfless Loving Service)

The great scientific achievements of modern science, and the money market economy of our society should not be considered as obstacles to spiritual development and self-realization. On the contrary, they must be utilized by people of good will to further the spiritual evolution and subsequently to achieve self-realization. This could become possible only if the views of humans can be changed. We should not remain the slaves of progress and material wealth anymore. On the contrary, progress and material wealth should be our servants. We are today in a stage where "the witchcraft novice" has not been able to control the forces he has created. He is over-powered and conducted by them.

The life of most living humans is concentrated only upon gaining material wealth, which according to them will secure all other sensual enjoyments. So for them a concentrated permanent material search is a vital necessity. However, psychological research has shown that those who are caught in the belief that the physical body is the focus of all pleasures in their lives along with money are usually the victims of depression, anxiety, unhappiness, and all psychological problems.

To those, the spiritual gate is momentarily closed. However, it remains open for those who are using their material wealth without any attachment and are sharing it by supporting some valuable socio-spiritual works. For those great souls, meditation becomes an easy task which leads to the divine while living in this vast, selfish, material world.

The businessmen and women, the medical doctors, the scientists, the artists, the professionals, the intellectuals, and the manual workers— should they be condemned to accede to the way which leads to spiritual evolution because of the busy activities? The science of yoga answers NO. On the contrary, there is a place in yoga for each and every one of those busy people.

Yoga will help them serve the public better (through Karma yoga) by performing conscientiously and honestly their jobs. By acting in this way, they will be happy and will live in peace. Usually the artists, the scientists, and the medical doctors are among the most loving, sensitive people. They will find in yoga a mirror in which they can take a better look at themselves in order to spread their warm beneficial feelings upon those who come in contact with them.

If a person, while living in society, honestly fulfills his or her social duty, if that person manifests an impersonal love in all the actions of life, and if the leisure time is used for the practice of Karma yoga and collective meditation, that person can accomplish the total spiritual evolution as well as the monk who is living in a solitary jungle cave. The noisy, agitated cities with all their material attractions should not divert the mind from internal search.

One must be able to isolate oneself from the noise and the crowd of modern life. One needs to follow the middle way traced by one of the greatest sages, Gautama Buddha, who incarnated on this planet more than 25 centuries ago. The way which the other great master, Jesus Christ, was shown when he said: "Give to Caesar the matter which belongs to him, and to God the Spirit." It is through karma yoga, unselfish services to all, and the disinterested action without the expectation of the fruit that one can achieve real love and self-realization.

This is a NEW AGE YOGA for suffering humanity. We all know that selfishness is the basic problem in this world and the main cause of all physical conflicts. If the NEW AGE KARMA YOGA can pacify our minds and soften our hearts, the world will then become a better place for all of us to live in peace during our short stay on this planet. The compassionate way of selfless service and divine love are the karma yoga way, which already has been shown to all by the great Master of Galilee. It is considered to be the way which will open the chakras of the heart for self-realization.

Karma yoga is the easiest way, which prepares a student for higher knowledge. It will purify the body and the mind. It will also develop the sensitivity of the heart, in order to understand and to feel better the descent of cosmic vibrations in the heart.

In fact, karma yoga is the first step of all other yoga disciplines. If you feel deep in your heart a desire to help without any condition, to serve whenever you get a chance to do so, then you are born to be happy and to taste the divine fruit of the cosmic world. Such unselfish desire will certainly lead you to the guru master, who will show you the way to self-realization in this very birth. We can say that the science of yoga opens to the sincere seeker the way to harmonious living, in which such a seeker is conscious of being useful to his or her brothers, and at the same time is feeling the spiritual progress towards the goal.

Can we dare to say that in this 21st century there are no other possible spiritual ways to salvation? From the social agitations we are observing all over the world, reported daily by the media, we can say that some powerful energies are at work on this planet and consequently in humans. From all sides, the stress is increasing upon a humanity in which two world wars have not been able to enlighten us upon the real sense of life and death. The necessity of spiritual development is registered in the projects of great beings who are responsible for the construction of the new age. Everywhere some spectacular changes of all kinds are succeeding each other at a great speed.

How would humanity be able to face the destiny of its future? How would it be able to choose between the spiritual light in a karma yoga or the materialistic darkness? Should it undergo the fate of Sodom and Gomorrah (Book of Genesis) or the vanished continent of Atlantis under the Ocean (in 355 BC)?

During the whole history of the world, the responsibility of each woman and man in her or his free will has never been as serious as it is today. It is for this reason that the great beings who are the guardians of humanity, and who are working on a superior level, have brought into the light of all the ancient science of yoga. If yoga is spreading more and more in the world, that is because it is a vital necessity for the cry of the soul, the body, and at the same time for the imperative actual global conjecture.

Finally, we hope that this verification will contribute and strengthen your efforts in yoga. Due to the well-known scientific and spiritual benefits of yoga, we can affirm that as yesterday, today, or tomorrow, the science of yoga will always help the sincere seeker to progress toward self-realization.

CHAPTER XIV

THE ACTION OF YOGA UPON THE ENTIRE
HUMAN COMPLEX SYSTEM

We have seen that the practice of the asanas has a powerful mechanical action upon the spinal column. Furthermore, we can see that the three combined disciplines of postures, breathing, and mental concentration also act upon the entire functions in the human complex system.

This complex action is produced for an important part through the ethereal body, which transfers the Pranic magnetic energy to the gross physical body. It is the prana, as previously stated, which through the nervous system and the sanguine current carries life to the cells and organs of the body.

To combine together the whole effects of yoga, we have not to neglect the unity and the complexity of the human body. The interdependence of the organs is the law. A human is an energy complex in which every center acts upon the other. Any disturbances somewhere affect the whole bodily system, and what we mean by human being is the whole organic life; that is, psychological, emotional, mental, and spiritual so closely bound. Let us now see the various beneficial effects produced by the practice of yoga.

EFFECTS UPON THE ARTICULATIONS
AND THE MUSCULAR SYSTEM

Besides the spinal column, the articulations and the muscles are also greatly affected by the asanas. For example, in Goraksasana and Padmasana, the articulation of the hips, the knees, and the ankles are also affected. From this, they will remain young. The blood is circulating well in the arteries, and the process of degeneration is retarded. With regular practice, any early sign of osteoarthritis or rheumatoid arthritis could be automatically regulated.

Most of the postures act upon the muscular system to vivify them and to maintain their elasticity. Some act upon the abdominal muscles and the major pectorals. Others affect the spinal and dorsal muscles, and some others work upon the lateral muscles of the trunk and the limbs muscles. All the muscles of the body are solicited by the whole yoga asanas. In this way, the muscular fibers maintain their vigor and elasticity until old age itself is delayed.

EFFECTS UPON THE DIGESTIVE SYSTEM

By the regular practice of yoga the digestive system should be working properly, with regular daily motion taking place. The pranayamas provoke an adequate activity of the diaphragm, which produces a continuous massage of the abdominal cavity. All the organs of this cavity are affected and vitalized.

Many asanas have also some powerful actions upon the organs. The liver, the pancreas, the stomach, the spleen, the intestines—all are solicited by the asanas. The secretions are improved, the sanguine irrigation is increased, stasis is reduced, nervous flux is circulating better, and the peristaltic movements are regularized.

The muscles of the abdominal strap, which play an essential role in the maintenance and the efforts of the internal organs, are strengthened at the same time by some asanas and deep breathing. The digestive transit is improved, and any constipation problem is normalized.

EFFECTS UPON THE CIRCULATORY
AND RESPIRATORY SYSTEM

First of all, the science of breathing deals with the respiratory function. The different techniques already described strengthen the lungs, develop their capacity, and increase the oxygenation of the blood. They also purify the respiratory channels and maintain the elasticity of the pulmonary alveolus. Some asanas irrigate the lungs with fresh blood and regenerate the tissues of the pulmonary lobules. Others work upon the respiratory channels—the nose, the throat, the pharynx, the larynx, the tonsils—and keep clean the gates where the air is flowing through. It is also known that the practice of pranayama can improve the negative conditions of asthma and early stage of emphysema.

Yoga is also very beneficial for the circulatory system. The slow, deep breathing and retention of the breath have a direct effect upon strengthening of the heart. With regular practice of pranayama the control of emotion becomes automatic, leading to a steady state of psychological wellbeing. Research shows that among regular practitioners of yoga, anxiety and depression are almost nonexistent.

EFFECTS UPON THE NERVOUS AND ENDOCRINE SYSTEM

The nervous and the endocrine system have a major responsibility in maintaining a healthy heart. They are interdependent upon each other. However, according to yogic knowledge, they also depend upon the condition of the vital or ethereal body from which they have received their energy supply (prana). It is by controlling those psychic centers or chakras, with the circulation of prana in the ethereal body that the sadhaka can master the health. The regular practice of yoga will certainly lead to this end.

Furthermore, some asanas also affect the nervous system directly. A combined practice of asanas, pranayamas, and mental concentration act upon the sympathetic system, which we know in psychology is responsible for the "fight or flight" response when a stressful or harmful attack is perceived. The nervous equilibrium is linked to the endocrinal equilibrium and the correct hormonal secretions of different glands, which condition a sound health.

The endocrine system consists of the pineal gland, the pituitary, the pancreas, the ovaries, the testes, the thyroid gland, the parathyroid glands, the hypothalamus, the gastrointestinal track, and the adrenal glands. Those glands are much affected with the yoga asanas, which usually act upon one or many of them. The asanas help in their correct irrigation and bring them vitality. Since the internal secretive glands formed one whole interdependent complex, the improvement of a gland s upon the entire glandular system. At the end, the result is sound health and complete recovery from diseases.

∾

LESSON 12   **PART 2**
THE ASANAS

THE COMPLETE WHEEL POSTURE (Purnachakrasana)
EXECUTION: Lying on the back, catch the legs and bend them as near as possible toward the buttocks, and then place both hands flat on the floor near the shoulders. Take a deep exhalation, and then lift up the body, while inhaling, with the help of the hands and the feet. Hold the breath along with the posture as long as you can. Come back slowly to the starting position in exhaling. Repeat two to three times the exercise, and then take a rest in Shavasana.

CONCENTRATION: Upon the throat center or the thyroid gland.

RESPIRATION: As indicated with the posture, but you can remain a longer time in the position when the body is in the curved position with straight arms, and then breathe normally.

THERAPEUTIC RESULTS: It brings suppleness to the lumbar region. It is also a great tonic for the muscles of the legs, the thighs, and the abdominals. It also irrigates the throat, the thyroid gland, and the head.

THE SHAKING POSTURE (Lolasana)
EXECUTION: Sit with crossed legs, just as in Padmasana (lotus posture), place hands flat on the floor, one on each side of the thighs. Take a deep inhalation and raise the body up. You are standing only on the hands. Hold the position with the breath as long as you can, and then come back down. Repeat the exercise three to four times, and then take rest.

CONCENTRATION: Upon the balance in the posture.

RESPIRATION: As indicated in the exercise, but you can also breathe normally to remain longer in the posture.

THERAPEUTIC RESULTS: It helps in the development of arm muscles, neck, and shoulder strength.

A VARIANT OF THE ROOSTER POSTURE (Kukutasana)
Remember that all these following postures are performed in the variant of Padmasana or Lotus Posture.

EXECUTION: Sit with crossed legs just as in the previous posture. The only difference in this posture is that the arms, instead of being outside of the thighs, are tight between the back leg muscles and the thighs. Take a deep inhalation and push up the body. Remain standing on the hands as long as you can.

CONCENTRATION: On the strength of the arms and the balance

RESPIRATION: Normal

RESULT: Same as in the previous exercise.

THE MOUNTAIN POSTURE (Parvatasana)

EXECUTION: Sit with crossed legs, enlace the fingers of both hands with each other, and turn the arms straight up. The palms of the hands are facing upward. First exhale, and then inhale while inclining the body on a straight line from right to left. On each side, hold the position with the breath for a few second. Keep swinging from right to left as many times you want, keeping the arms straight.

CONCENTRATION: On the movement of the posture

RESPIRATION: As described with the exercise

RESULTS: Same as in the previous one, but it adds more elasticity to the trunk and the shoulder muscles.

VERTICAL LOTUS POSTURE (Urdhvapadmasana)

EXECUTION: From the sitting of the lotus position, lay flat on the back with the arms straight alongside the body. Take a deep inhalation with the help of the hands, rise up to the vertical the trunk with crossed legs. The whole body is now resting in the vertical position on the shoulders and the neck. The hands are placed behind the trunk to support the body, and the elbows are on the floor. Breathe normally and remain in the position as long as you can, and then come back and take a rest.

CONCENTRATION: Upon the spinal column at the cervical region.

RESPIRATION: Slow and regular.

THERAPEUTIC RESULTS: It strengthens the shoulder muscles, the spinal column, and nourishes the thyroid gland and the brain.

THE LOTUS IN HALASANA (Shirshasprushta-Padmasana)

EXECUTION: From the lotus posture, lay flat on the back, the hands placed alongside the body. Take a deep inhalation and stretch up the body with the help of the elbows and the hands. Keep on stretching until the knees of the crossed legs get as close as possible to the floor. Hold the posture and breathe normally. The head is now reverse backward on the floor.

CONCENTRATION: Upon the spinal column at the cervical region.

RESPIRATION: Slow and normal.

RESULTS: Same as in the previous variant, but more powerful.

ABDOMINAL RETRACTION IN LOTUS
(Uddiyana Bandha-Padmasana)

If you have mastered the Padmasana, you then will be able to perform this *kriya*, or *Bandha*.

EXECUTION: Sit in Padmasana with the hands resting lightly on the knees. Take a deep inhalation. While helping yourself with the pressure on the knees, hollow to the maximum the belly. Hold the Bandha, or the lock, for a few seconds with the breath retention, and then exhale while giving up the abdominal contraction, and then breathe normally.

CONCENTRATION: Upon the exercise.

RESULTS: It gives internal massage to the abdomen and strengthens the cavities.

HALF TIED LOTUS POSTURE (Ardha Baddha Padmasana)

EXECUTION: Sit in Padmasana, and place the right arm behind the back and try to catch the left toe with the heel of the foot pressing the left side of the belly, bent forward to the left, while raising your left arm up in the air. Hold the position for a few seconds, and then reverse the position on the other side. When bending forward, first take a deep inhalation and exhale while holding the posture, and then breathe normally.

CONCENTRATION: Upon the spleen, when the heel of the foot is pressing the left side of the belly, and on the liver when the heel is pressing the right side of the belly.

THERAPEUTIC RESULTS: It gives massage to the liver, the spleen, strengthens the shoulder muscles, and works more upon the knee joints.

COMPLETE TIED LOTUS POSTURE (Baddha Padmasana)
EXECUTION: From the previous variant of the half tied lotus posture, instead of straightening out the arm, enlace both hands behind the back and try to catch both big toes, when bending forward. If not possible, just rest the hands on the thighs while bending forward and breathe normally. In performing this posture, each time you bend, go to the left and alternate to the right.

CONCENTRATION: It is the same as indicated in the previous posture. If the heels of the feet can touch the sides of the belly, focus as in the previous posture on the spleen or the liver, depending on which side you are on.

BREATHING: Normal.

RESULTS: The same as stated in the previous asana.

THE SCIENCE OF BREATHING (Pranayama)

THE FEEDING PRANAYAMA

Sit in the lotus posture or any comfortable posture, take a deep inhalation. Bend forward the head and press the chin tightly against the chest while holding on to your breath. This retention must be very long. When the tension has become uncomfortable, exhale slowly and breathe normally. Repeat the full exercise 3 to 6 times.

RESULTS: This pranayama has a powerful mental and psychological effect, mostly on the mind of those who practice meditation.

DOUBLE RETENTION PRANAYAMA

EXECUTION: Sit in any comfortable posture, take a deep complete inhalation. Hold the breath with full lungs. Exhale and retain the breath with empty lungs before taking another inhalation.

This pranayama is characterized by the two retentions. The first one with full lungs is called *interior calix*. The second retention with empty lungs is called *exterior calix*.

RHYTHM: The traditional rhythm used for this pranayama is: 1-4-2-2. If the inhalation lasts 3 seconds, the first retention will be of 12 seconds, the exhalation of 6 seconds, and the second retention of 6 seconds. In some cases, the rhythm of 1-4-2-4 can also be used, but somewhat more difficult. You should of course gradually increase the length of the retention.

CONCENTRATION: Upon the exercise.

RESULTS: The results are psychic and help in the practice of advanced yoga. *N.B. – This pranayama can really be useful only for the student who is interested in Higher yoga.*

❧

LESSON 12   **PART 3**

HIGHER YOGA
The Way to Immortality

Every day people are dying, leaving this world after a short stay, full of unhappiness. For many people, life itself is like a valley of tears. One cannot say that one is feeling happy and content all the time. Every day some new creatures are taking birth to replace those who have left. In this way, the cycle of birth and death is moving permanently at full speed. At the death of a loved relative or a friend we feel grief, and for a moment we have the impression that the Creator is unfair to take away from us our beloved. However, when a new baby comes into the home of a couple, it is the contrary which happens. Everybody feels happy with a lot of cheer. During this moment, they glorify the Creator and thank Him for His mercy and His greatness.

Why should we take birth for a short time and die again? Is it really the divine will of the Creator? Can this yoga really help us to stop the cycle of birth and death through a final complete liberation?

According to the esoteric science of yoga, the cycle of birth and death is a process of evolution. Every time a human being incarnates on earth, the quality of his or her seed is different from the previous one. We can try to understand this mystery if we can take a look at us in this world. Out of the 7.4 billion human beings living on this planet today, each one of us is different and unique, although we all have the same internal organs, the same life principle, the same color of blood, and the same color of seed. Only the skin complexion is different, due to different races. However, our spiritual feelings are different, intellectual understandings are different, and we all feel some differences in our relation with Mother Nature (between the microcosm and the macrocosm). Can you tell why a person is interested in a deep search for his or her spiritual inner being, and why his or her brother or a friend is interested only in lower worldly pleasure and has no feelings for any spiritual search?

Well, the yogic literatures tell us that it is a question of quality of the seed in which everyone has been developed. A yogi or a great spiritual being is the product of a highly developed seed, which has undergone different processes of mutations during many previous births.

One has to come again and again on earth until one seed becomes pure light, and such a seed will give birth to a pure physical body which shall never die or be reborn again. For this divinely purified seed the cycle of birth and dead has ended. This theory is quite scientific and it explains the material, intellectual, and spiritual inequality between humans.

From this theory, we cannot blame the Creator (who is always neutral) for taking away the life of our beloved, which apparently he has given. We can understand that the Creator is almost comparable to the sun, which is spreading its warm rays upon all: the rich, the poor, the criminal, and the saint. We can also understand that from that point of view, everyone has his or her chance one day to reach perfection, after a total purification of all negative karma.

The Creator is so perfect in His will that He has not forgotten His created beings. He has endowed us with the divine spark in us to light up again and awaken us from our long worldly dream, which has stopped our spiritual evolution.

Through the holistic yoga, which is the heritage of humans and the most natural science, this spiritual device can be set up into action. After suffering a lot during the purification process of many births, a great soul comes and starts taking interest in yoga. Such a soul will be open-minded. His or her view of God will be deeply hidden in the heart, and they won't be in any temple, church, or religion. Since such soul is already the product of a superior seed, the prejudices of a hypocritical society will never be his concern. Yoga, which will make him feel the divine manifestation in his own flesh, will be his only true religion. Having such a divine feeling inside oneself will certainly lead to the divine universal love of Christ. All the teachings we have given in these lessons can help sincere seekers to free themselves from further physical or moral sufferings, and eventually achieve final liberation from birth and death.

Furthermore, to purify the remaining impurities in the physical body, there is no better therapy than the yoga asanas. To remove the last impurities of the blood which come from the seed, there is not a better therapy than the pranayamas. To develop higher spiritual grades in the mind, there is no better instrument than the meditation. Finally, to achieve self-realization in this very birth, there is no better discipline than the holistic yoga knowledge.

Throughout these simple yoga lessons, we have drawn your attention about a deep hidden secret inside of you, which is your own Divine heritage. If the positive cosmic forces have directed you towards this secret, know that for sure it is not a hazard. From this revelation, you will have the opportunity to explore your inspirations, which some day will lead you to the discovery of your own self.

CHAPTER XV

SYNTHESIS OF THE HOLISTIC YOGA

T hroughout this book, we have showed the commonly known technique of yoga called hatha yoga. It has been stated that it is through this hatha yoga, which deals with the physical body, that one can eventually reach the mind and realize the self. However, how about all the other kinds of yoga? Are they inferior to hatha yoga? Or can they also lead a seeker to self-realization?

To those questions a sadhaka may be confused and find it difficult to decide which yoga is suitable to her needs. Besides the name hatha yoga, we usually hear many other names along with yoga, such as bhakti yoga, gyana yoga, karma yoga, raja yoga, kriya yoga, kundalini yoga, mantra yoga, nada yoga, hamsa yoga, shaktipata yoga, and purna yoga, etc. In fact, yoga is only one. All those different labels are only means to explain different techniques to realize the unity of yoga. Before a sadhaka can complete the final stage of yoga, she has to go through different yoga techniques. It was for this reason that the yoga masters had invented many different names to explain better the deep yoga science.

It is in the same way when we say "food", the word *food* means every kind of nourishment which gives strength to the body and keeps it healthy. Many different names are used under the word *food*, such as rice, peas, vegetable, cheese, milk, meat, eggs, flour, etc. But can we say that meat is food and vegetables are not? Or dare we assert that meat is a superior food to vegetables or the contrary? It depends on the organism which is taking these different diets. But the goal of the food is to nourish the body and to keep it alive.

Furthermore, we cannot say that any particular form of yoga is superior to another. Only the technique used by the aspirant can make that person feel whether this form of yoga is suitable or not, or probably lead to the desired goal of self-realization.

The word 'yoga' is so vast and deep that if different sub-titles were not added to it, it would have been very difficult to understand the idea of it. To explain better the yogic idea, we can say that it is just like different subjects one has to learn in school. In order to graduate, one has to have knowledge of all of the required subjects in the syllabus. None of the prescribed subjects is useless; however, they all will lead to the goal of graduation. Among these different appellations of yoga, we will study six of them and will try to arrive at the conclusion of the holistic yoga. They are: karma yoga, bhakti yoga, shaktipata yoga, kundalini yoga, raja yoga, and purna yoga.

The ancient yogi masters had detailed the yoga subject to their pupils to help them to succeed quicker in their goal. Usually, the first yoga which will be taught by the master is karma yoga. What is karma yoga?

KARMA YOGA - It deals with loving, unselfish services to others. Suppose there is a yogi who has become enlightened and has reached the goal of self-realization, with the possession of divine power. If such powerful yogi has not practiced karma yoga, he or she will think of dominating the world instead of showing the way to others. Fortunately, the Supreme Lord is so rightful and perfect, and will not allow such yogi who has not practiced karma yoga to realize the Self.

Karma yoga is the way that purifies the body and the mind. A selfish person cannot become a yogi. When you do a good action to others, the fruit of it automatically comes to you, though it was unexpected. Suppose you witnessed an accident on the road; two children are the victims, and nobody else is around but you. Instead of going your way, you stopped as the good Samaritan, you called the authorities, and you gave the victims first aid. Later on, you came to know that they are safe because of your good intervention. The childrens' parents and friends are looking for you to congratulate you. This is the automatic, unexpected fruit of your good action. However, way before this result, you were feeling happy at doing a good action to others. What you have done is a karma yoga, which has upgraded your heart.

Many will come to yoga and wish to obtain good health, happiness, and yoga siddhis (power). However, morally they are not prepared, and there is no place for love in their heart. For such aspirants, unless they can develop the will to practice a very active karma yoga, failure in yoga will always be nearer than success.

Usually the miserable people with constant negative thoughts and who are suffering from various physical illnesses are mostly those who have identified themselves with material wealth. They think only of themselves and their own family. If they start practicing karma yoga, they will at once notice some improvements in their health, because the physical body is connected with the feelings. Good or bad feelings have an impact upon the physical body and the mind. The ancient yogis were well aware of this fact; that is why they had prescribed the practice of karma yoga.

BHAKTI YOGA – This is the yoga of divine love and spiritual devotion. Usually when we talk about self-realization, behind it there is a feeling of self-superiority. In the yoga scriptures there are some tales about yogis who had become so powerful that they had threatened the peace of the kingdom of Brahma the Creator.

The ego in man is the biggest obstacle to self-realization. A sadhaka who thinks that he or she can get enlightened with the self-power is mistaken. The sadhaka first has to purify the ego through bhakti yoga. In this yoga the sadhaka does not have the impression of doing anything. She just surrenders the will to the divine will. Through satsang, she sings the divine name of the Lord and the whole vibration of love is flowing in the heart. She sees the Lord everywhere and in everyone. She remains intoxicated with divine joy. The practice of bhakti yoga develops the feelings and the idea of universal love.

How can a yogi become enlightened without practicing this yoga? Bhakti yoga is the key which opens the door to higher regions of yoga. A bhakti yogi has so much divine love in the heart that he could never disregard anyone or feel any superiority of ideas. You can feel that this yoga is also related to karma yoga. If there is selfless action, there is automatically bhakti (love). If there is love, the power of the ego is subdued, and there is a greater need to serve than of being served.

Some aspirants are naturally born with a great amount of bhakti, or devotional love, in their heart. They are the mystics, the universalist thinkers. Wherever they are, in open nature or in their rooms, they always have a feeling of divine contact. However, those seekers who are not gifted with the bhakti quality have to develop it through practice. The spiritual songs practiced in churches, temples, ashrams, and yoga centers are means of bhakti yoga. They attract divine vibrations, which transform slowly the heart and the mind of the sadhaka

SHAKTIPATA YOGA – This yoga is the transmission of invisible flux into the subtle body of an aspirant. The word *shakti* means force or energy, and *Ppata* means to impart. After the impartation of pranic energy by a siddha master to a disciple, he or she begins at once to feel the manifestation of prana in the body. The sadhaka's body becomes just like if it is possessed by a spirit. She begins to sing, to dance, to perform various yoga asanas, and to weep. She is overjoyed with the newborn divine shakti, and is feeling strong. To be fit for shakti-pata diksha, the aspirant has first to prepare the heart. This work can be done only through karma and bhakti yoga. On the other hand, you can understand that karma yoga and shaktipata yoga are related to each other.

In shaktipata yoga, the practice of devotional songs, which are done in bhakti yoga will automatically come out. Same as the asanas performed in hatha yoga will also be performed by the energy of shakti-pata. In fact, without shakti-pata, which raises the pranic energy in the body, real understanding of esoteric yoga is not possible. The awakening of prana is the fruit of bhakti and karma yoga.

If a sadhaka receives shaktipata without first practicing bhakti and karma yoga, the result will be that disturbances will arise in the body. She will be so much overpowered by the awakening pranic energy that fear will arise in the mind, and she will give up the yoga practice. She will be under the impression that an evil spirit has entered her body, and the Master who has acted upon her is not a holy person. Therefore, she will seek elsewhere for exorcism!

This is the danger for an impure seeker whose mind is dominated by evil thoughts and selfish motives. A wise guru will never think of initiating such a seeker into shaktipata yoga, because doing so will be more harmful to her than beneficial.

It is just like putting a young child alone behind the wheel of a car in busy street. The child may not only kill himself, but the life and properties of others are threatened. Before stepping up into Sshaktipata yoga, the heart and the mind must be purified by many years of regular practice of bhakti and karma yoga. Without the fulfillment of the rules of these two different yoga techniques, one should not venture in the field of Sshaktipata yoga. From this analytic study, you can understand that as far as holistic development is concerned, karma yoga, bhakti yoga, and shaktipata yoga cannot be separated.

KUNDALINI YOGA – This yoga is quite popular among seekers for siddhis, or occult powers. *Kundalini* is a very big word used by many famous yogi masters. Mostly in every book on yoga, this subject is discussed. Since kundalini is symbolized as the goddess of divine power and knowledge, so any guru who can elaborate on this topic is regarded as someone in possession of divine power, or the *siddhis*. In fact, what is kundalini?

In the yoga Upanishad, kundalini has been described in a symbolic and esoteric way. The yoga masters by their wisdom have always wanted to keep this knowledge secret. However, at the same time they wished to inspire the sincere seekers, so they had described esoterically the kundalini yoga in the yogic scriptures. Unfortunately, many learned men have mistaken kundalini for a mysterious serpent which is supposed to enter the body of the sadhaka while in meditation. Some yogis have prescribed to their student different techniques to arise the kundalini. All are talking about it, but very few really know what it is all about. All these interests are generated around kundalini because its awakening is supposed to confer some occult powers known as siddhis.

Kundalini cannot be awakened without shaktipata. Its awakening is the result of successful practice of shaktipata yoga. From this statement, you can understand that a selfish sadhaka who is after occult powers cannot succeed in kundalini yoga. You can also understand why all are talking about this subject, and why very few can get access to it. The heart must first be purified through Karma and Bhakti yoga. Complete renunciation of material wealth and even of the occult powers is the basic condition of the awakening of kundalini. This yoga is only for the one who is after liberation (moksha), the one who wishes to free himself or herself from further sufferings in this very birth. She alone is fit to understand all the secrets of kundalini. Since she does not have any worldly desires, not even for name and fame, why then should she speak or describe the technique of kundalini? Here again, you can understand why the ancient yogis could not give away openly the process of kundalini yoga. It is a personal and incommunicable experience reserved only for those great gifted mystics. Those who really know about it will always keep the secret, because its disclosure could only shock and expose to danger the unfit seeker who may try to awake it.

The beauty of yoga is that it is a self-experimental science. That is, for one to really understand the psychological, spiritual, and physical effects of yoga, one must be willing to experiment within one's own body. To draw an analogy about honey, if someone asks you what the taste of honey is, what can you say: just "sweet?" However, the word *sweet* does not really explain the taste of honey. The one who really wants to know the taste of honey must do a self-taste.

So before thinking about kundalini yoga, the body, the mind, and the heart must be purified, and this process can occur only through karma yoga, bhakti yoga, and shaktipata yoga practice. Once more, you understand that kundalini yoga is also related with the other yoga techniques previously described. It is in the same way that all the internal organs in the body are related with each other and are necessary for the proper functioning of the entire bodily complex. You may be able to live without a lung or a kidney, and in that case, you will be considered as a handicap. However, you cannot live without a heart. In yoga, kundalini represents the heart. You may practice hatha yoga with all the other yogas, but you cannot practice kundalini yoga without first purifying the mind, the intellect, and the body with the help of other yoga techniques.

RAJA YOGA - The word *raja* means *royal*. So, raja yoga is the royal way which leads to salvation. This yoga is also very popular. It is found in every book on yoga, and all the sadhakas are very fond of this word. When you tell someone that you are practicing raja yoga, that makes you feel important and gives you a divine personality, but are you sure that you are really practicing raja yoga?

Let us see in detail what raja yoga is. According to the Yoga Upanishads, raja yoga is the fruit of the complete mastery over the physical body through hatha yoga. The mastery of the asanas does not mean that one has mastered hatha yoga. We already have dealt plenty with hatha yoga in twelve lessons of this book, but to better explain raja yoga, we have to take another deep look at it. The seven main chakras in the body we have studied must be fully developed in order to master hatha yoga. Each chakra gives a special control over a particular region of the body. For example, the mastery over *Anahat* chakra confers the control of the heart region. There are two main vital air currents in the body, which the yogi has to master. They are known as *prana wayu* and *apana wayu*. Prana wayu regularizes the breath circulation which flows upward, and apana wayu regularizes the breath circulation which flows downward. It is also responsible for the elimination of urine and for bowel movements. There is always a fight in the body between these two vital airs

The fight is increased after the awakening of kundalini shakti. Of course, the energy of kundalini wants to pierce the chakras and to go upwards, while apana wants to bring it back down. Every time kundalini from Muladhara chakra rises up to a higher chakra—for example, Anahat—apana wayu will pull her back to where she was. It is just like a bird attached to a tree with a long rope. Every time he tries to fly in the air, the rope will bring him back down. When a yogi is able to control the two *wayus*, at that time the goddess Kundalini will be able to sit permanently wherever she wants, in any chakra, without fear of being pulled down by apana. This is the most difficult task, and without it no real Raja yoga practice is possible. It is the full development of the chakra which will lead to the unification of prana with apana wayu.

Before the awakening of kundalini shakti, the chakras were considered virtual in the body. After the awakening, they became real, but in an embryonic stage only. Their developments require not only a lifetime of regular yoga practice, but also many births. That is why it is stated in the yogic scriptures that Self-realization, which means full development of the human body, requires many births.

Suppose you have been practicing yoga for many years. You were fortunate enough to have your prana shakti awakened, but the body died without reaching the final goal. In your next birth you will come back with all the qualities you had gained in order to continue the work and nothing will be lost. In your new body, the task to develop the chakras will be much easier and raja yoga will become possible.

As it has been taught in one of the lessons, the chakras are psychic centers or knots, which give control to the part of the body related to each chakra. In Rraja yoga, during meditation the sadhaks have to focus inside each chakra in order to raise up kundalini in the body. When in meditation, they have to study the details of each chakra, the shape, the color, and the intensity of each light they see within the chakras. The mind must be so busy with the intensity of the meditation that it becomes absorbed in the chakras. This is called raja yoga. However, to arrive at such a stage, karma yoga, bhakti yoga, shaktipata yoga, and kundalini yoga must be previously practiced. Again, it is understood that without the mastery of those stages, the practice of raja yoga is impossible.

We often hear that term *transcendental meditation* used by some yogis who are after name and fame to attract people. It is supposed to confer some siddhis (miraculous powers) and lead to peace and salvation. This transcendental meditation is nothing else but the process of raja yoga. The word *transcendental* means *ordinary human experiences,* and according to the yoga Upanishads, a yogi in transcendental meditation, or raja yoga, has gone above the mind stuff, and when the moment arrives to come out of it, he will come enlightened with siddhis or divine miraculous power.

We heard that there are several thousand ordinary men and women in the world who are practicing transcendental meditation. Then are they all enlightened, able to levitate, with real siddhis as the propaganda claimed? Do not kid yourself; a sincere sadhaka will not absorb this crap. If it was so easy, all would have been able to fly in the air like the birds, and remain anyway conditioned mortal beings. Raja yoga is a stage of yoga reserved only for the sadhaka who is after salvation (mukti). The one who is after name, fame, and material wealth can only enjoy the name of raja yoga, not the divine experiences. Again, after all of these explanations, you can understand that raja yoga is also related to the other yoga techniques and cannot be separated.

PURNA YOGA - The name of this yoga is usually found in the esoteric yoga Upanishads. The word *purna* means 'complete.' A purna yogi is the one who has mastered prana and apana wayu with all the yoga techniques, and who has reached the state of *nirvikalpa samadhi,* or liberation (mukti) with divine body. The adept of this yoga is the one who has received shaktipata initiation and has awakened the kundalini power. There is no need of telling anything further about purna yoga. It is all the yoga techniques in one, and this is the holistic yoga.

After all those comparative studies of yoga, you must be convinced by now about its unity. The moment one steps into the study of yoga, one is dealing with one subject—the holistic yoga. You may not be able to reach right away certain stages of yoga due to circumstances, environmental obstacles, and your own disposition. However, the door will remain open for you as you are developing.

Furthermore, as you can see, no yoga is superior to the other one. A sadhaka should not think that the yoga taught by his or her guru is superior to the one taught by another guru. Only ignorance could create such thoughts in the mind. The goal of all yogas is to master the mind and to reach the transcendental state of samadhi (mindless state).

However, we can say that certain techniques of yoga could be more efficient than others, and will lead quicker to the goal. As you know, from the suburban area of a big city, there are different means of transportation to reach the city. One can go by train, bus, car, cycle, or even on foot. The time to arrive in the city will depend on the transportation means which has been used. Suppose you are practicing hatha yoga alone with the help of books; you cannot expect to progress safely and at the same speed as if you had received shaktipata from a guru. However, if you are following the moral rules of yoga, and practicing honestly, you may one day find the guidance of a master. This will depend on your own karma. But shaktipata yoga has the power to burn all your past and present karma, and finally gets you closer to the goal in this very birth. So the superiority of yoga is only in the technique used.

Now, let us see how to choose a yoga model. After this comparative study of all the yoga techniques, some sadhakas may find difficulties in the choice of a suitable yoga path, since we said that they all are one. Some others may desire to practice shaktipata yoga, or to sit and wait for a guru to initiate them in the proper yoga path. What you need is a proper understanding of yourself, and a great desire to improve your health and to solve all your personal problems. If these basic conditions are met, the choice should not be that much difficult. Yes, yoga is one, but different techniques must be practiced at different stages before realizing its unity.

The first choice which is valid for all is the yoga which takes care of the health of the physical body, which is hatha yoga. Without a healthy, strong physical body, the mental cannot vibrate positively with the physical. Therefore, a desire to practice karma yoga through services to others will remain ineffective. As far as shaktipata and kundalini yoga are concerned, only sadhakas with strong permanent health can undertake such delicate work. In fact, hatha yoga is the basic yoga which prepares the physical and the mental for the practice of different yoga techniques. Without the legs you cannot walk, you can only crawl, and by crawling, it will take you much time and with great difficulty to go wherever you wish to go.

Without hatha yoga, the others will be much more difficult to reach. There are some yogis who, because of ignorance, neglect the physical body. They think of reaching samadhi through the practice of mantra yoga alone, or bhakti, or jnana yoga. What happens is this—during all their lives they are suffering with all kind of diseases just like ordinary people. They have to keep taking daily medicines to bring relief to the body, and finally they die after great mental and physical suffering. Then how can we say they had a happy life, and peacefully they have reached salvation?

Concerning salvation, you will find this statement in all the yoga Upanishads "For one to be called a jivanmukta or a liberated soul, all diseases must have vanished in the body, it must become pure light burning in the fire of yoga." From this quotation, it is understood that the diseases are the enemies of yoga. However, to vanquish the enemy, one has to use the weaponry of all the yoga techniques.

It really does not matter the name you wish to give to a particular yoga you are practicing; the idea is to live a peaceful, harmonious life within yourself, and to leave this world after fulfilling all the duties of this present birth. Remember that death is just like a long dream. In sleeping dream, all the desires of the wakeful state are still with you and they cannot be controlled by the power of your will. Suppose in the sleeping state you dream of someone who is taking away your money right in the room where you are sleeping. Your subconscious may awake you to protect your belonging. However, in the death dream such impression will only retard your process of evolution and increase the suffering of unsatisfied desires. Because the body is dead, so the subconscious cannot awake you to satisfy your desires by ascertaining that your belonging are still with you. A combined practice of all the yoga techniques will prepare the mind, the body, and the subconscious to enjoy a peaceful life in the dream state as well as after the death of the body.

GLOSSARY

The Sanskrit words are given in a very simple transcription to help the readers to pronounce the word correctly.

The *a,i*, and *u* vowels. The Sanskrit has these three earliest and most universal vowels of Indo-European language, in both short and long form. That is *a* and *aa*, *i* and *ii*, *u* and *uu*. They are to be pronounced in the "continental or Italian" manner as in *far* or *father*, *pin* and *pique*, pull and *rule*. *C* is pronounced *ch*. *J* is pronounced *jh*.

AJNA: Psychic center situated in the middle of the eyebrows.

ANAHATA: Psychic center situated in the chest at the heart region.

APANA WAYU: One of the five life-winds in the body, which is responsible for all downwards work of the air performed in the body.

ASANA: Posture performed by the yogis.

BHANDHA: Muscular contraction.

BHAKTI: Devotional spiritual love.

BRAHMA: The Supreme Creator (God).

BRAHMAN or BRAHMIN: Hindu priest belonging to the superior caste in Hinduism.

CHAKRA: Psychic or energetic center located in different parts in the ethereal body.

DARSHANA: Philosophical systems or point of views. In orthodox Hinduism there are six main Darshans: Samkhya, Yoga, Vedanta, Niyaya, Mimamsa, and Vaisheshika.

FAKIR: An ascetic or mendicant with wonder power.

DIKSHA: Initiation given by the guru.

GUNA: An ingredient or constituent of Nature – anyone of the three qualities of Nature pervading all created things. They are: Satwa, Rajas, Tamas.

GURU: Spiritual Master; a guide who confers initiation.

GYANA yoga: The yoga of knowledge – Through it, one has to use the intellect as a mean to achieve Self-realization.

HAMSA: Individual soul.

HATHA YOGA: Union of the body with the Spirit by the practice of specific physical postures – Mixture of positive and negative energies of the body.

IDA: Psychic channel situated on the left side of the body.

JIVAMUKTI: Liberated soul.

KARMA: Positive or negative effects of whatever action performed in this birth or previous ones.

KRISHNA: Divine incarnation in Hinduism.

KRIYA: Symbolic gestures, cleansing process – esoteric actions performed by the limbs of the body.

KUMBHAKA: Breath retention in respiratory exercises.

KUNDALINI: Divine energy sleeping at the Muladhara chakra between the Sacrum and the genital.

MANIPURA CHAKRA: Psychic energy center situated at the navel region.

MANTRA: Hermetic word given to the disciple by the guru during initiation, to chant or to repeat for spiritual advancement.

MAYA: Illusion – an invisible power which keep dominating the mind and makes it adopt the unreal as real.

MUDRA: Symbolic gestures performed by the yogi in order to control positive and negative energies in the body.

MUKTI: Liberation – a state beyond birth and death.

MULADHARA: Psychic center situated between the sacrum and the genital.

MOKSHA: Salvation or Liberation.

NADI: Psychic channel in which subtle energy circulates.

NADA: Mystic sound felt inside the body.

NIYAMA: First part of the moral rules and discipline prescribed by the yoga science (Yama is the second part).

OM: Cosmic sound intoned as a Mantra during meditation.

PANDIT: Learned person well acquainted with yogic scriptures.

PATANJALI: A well-known author of the yoga aphorism, which believed to have lived in the second century (B.C.).

PINGALA: Psychic channel situated on the right side of the body.

PRANA WAYU: Vital air or life principal in the body.

PURNA yoga: holistic or complete yoga.

RAJASIC: Element of passion (see Guna).

RAJA YOGA: A royal yoga, which deals with concentration and meditation.

RISHI: Sage or great yoga master.

SADHAKA: Spiritual seeker or an advanced yoga student.

SAHASRARA or SAHASRADAL: The highest energy center on top of the head – a symbolic lotus with a thousand petals situated at the top of the head.

SAMADHI: A transcendental state which occurs during the practice of meditation.

SATSANGA: Meeting of seekers or devotees during which spiritual practices, devotional songs, and meditations are performed.

SATVIC or SATWIC: Quality of purified element (see Guna).

SHAKTI: Sleeping spiritual energy virtual in every human being.

SHARNAGATI: Self-surrender to the divine power within.

SHASTRA: Yogic scriptures.

SHISYA: Yoga student or disciple.

SHIVA: Mythical Hindu gods which are supposed to guide and protect the yogis.

SIDDHA: Perfect being, a realized soul.

SIDDHI: Miraculous power.

SHUSHUMNA: The main psychic channel in the body.

SUTRA: Aphorism, short yoga verses.

SVADHISTHANA: Psychic center or chakra situated below the navel region.

TAMASIC: A lethargic state or quality (see Guna).

UPANISHAD: Yogic scripture.

VEDA: Compiled spiritual materials which reveal the Brahmanic tradition.

SWAMI: Indian ascetic or an initiated person into a religious order.

SADHU: Mendicant ascetic.

VEDANTA: One of the three great Hindu's philosophical system.

VISHNU: Mythical Hindu god; the second person in the Brahmanic trinity.

VISHUDDHA: Psychic center situated at the throat region.

YAMA: Second part of the moral rules and discipline prescribed by the yoga science (Niyama is the first part).

YOGA: An ancient psycho-physical discipline first practiced in India thousands of years ago. Its aim is to unite the body and the mind with the Cosmic.

YOGI: Adept of the science of yoga.

REFERENCES CITED

Arundale, G.S. (1974). <u>Kundalini: An Occult Experience:</u> Madras, 1974.

Ayyangar, G.R. <u>The Yoga Upanishads:</u> Original translation of 20 Yoga Upanishads from Sanskrit, available on Hinduism E. Books.

Bess-Boss, A., Edelberg, D.(2009). <u>The Everything Digestive Health Book: What you Need to Know to Eat Well, be Healthy, and Feel Great.</u>

Bevalkar, S.K. (2006). <u>Vedanta Philosophy</u>: Jain Publishing Company, Victoria, Canada.

Bryant, W.W. (1918). <u>Men of Science, Galileo:</u> Society for Promoting Christian Knowledge, London,

Collison, D. (2006). <u>If the Hunsa People Could Live to 100 + Years, So Can We:</u> The Collison Newsletter (October, 20016).

Cramer, G.D., Darby, S.A. (2013). <u>Clinical Anatomy Spine, Spinal Cord, and Ans.:</u> Elsevier Health Science 3rd Edition, Cambridge, MA.

Emery, J. (2014), <u>The Anatomy of the Developing Lung:</u> Butterworth Heinement International Medical Publication.

Folgert, T. (2001). <u>"Quantum Shamantum: Discovery 22 :37-43, Nothing is Solid & Everything is Energy:</u> Scientific Explain.

Gevitz, N. (2004). <u>The Dos Osteopathic Medicine in America:</u> John Hopkins University Press, Baltimore, Maryland.

Gomez, M. (1987). <u>The Dawning of Theosophical Movement:</u> Quest Book, Wheaton, IL.

Hardward, R., Miller S., & Vasta, R. (2008). <u>Child Psychology; Development in a Changing Society</u>: Publisher Wiley, Hoboken, New Jersey, 5th Edition. Win Publishing, El Monte, California.

Johnson, L.R. (2003). <u>Essential Medical Physiology 3rd Edition:</u> Elsevier Academic Press, Cambridge, MA.

Johnson, L.R. (2013). <u>Gastro-intestinal Physiology, Mosby Physiology Monogram Series, 8th Edition:</u> Elsevier Health Science Academic Press, Cambridge, MA.

Misra, V. (1974). <u>Patanjali Yoga Sutras With the Commentary of Vyasa and the Gloss of Vachaspati Misra:</u> AMS Press, New York.

Mookerjee, A. (1982). <u>Kundalini, the Arousal of the Inner Energy:</u> Destiny Book, Rochester, Vermont.

Morrison, W.A. (2015). Synovial Fluid Analysis: Health line, December, 14, 2015.

Prabhupada, Swami, (1970). : The Vedanta Academi, gurukula).

Roth, S. M. (2006). Why Does Lactic Build-up in Muscles? And Why Does it Cause Soreness? Scientific American Jan. 23. 2016.

Ryan, J. (1995, 2000). Little Girls in Pretty Boxes: Warner Book, New York.

Satchidananda, S. (1978). The Yoga Sutra of Patanjali: Holistic Yoga Publication, Yoga Ville, Virginia.

Sing, P. (1914). Hatha Yoga Pradipika: Original Translation from Sanskrit: Panini office, Allahabad, India.

Spivey, N. (2012). The Ancient Olympics: Oxford University Press. New York.

Schaeffer, M.R., Mendonca, C.T., Levangie, M.C. Anerson, R.E., Taissalo, T. Jensen, D. (2014). Physiological Mechanisms of Sex Differences in Exertional Dyspnea: Role of Neural Respiratory Motor Drive: Experimental Physiology Volume 99, issue 2, G. 427-441.

The Bible: King James Version, Published, in 1611.

Vasu. C. (1979). Gheranda Samahita : Original text, translated from Sanskrit: Shri Satguru Publication, Delhi, India.

Vasu C. Siva Samhita: Original translation from Sanskrit: Shri Satguru Publication, Delhi, India.

Xinnong, C, Deng, L. (2000). Chinese Acupuncture and Moxibustion: Publisher: China Book and Periodical, Inc.

About the Author

Lauture Massac, Ph.D. is a clinical psychologist, with specialization in chemical dependency. He is licensed in the states of California and Tennessee. He has over 25 years of experience in working in mental health settings. Through his yoga knowledge, he has developed indigenous methods to treat patients, and to empower them with self-knowledge to resolve their psychological and mental health issues. He is a rare psychologist with a practical package of Eastern and Western philosophy knowledge to treat patients, and to inspire self-seekers to find the missing peace within.

Dr. Massac, also known as Yogi Darshan Muni, his initiated name given to him by his late great master guru Swami Shri Kripalu. Before becoming a psychologist, he studied yoga in India in different yoga schools. Among them is the famous Lonavala Yoga Institute in Poona, India, where he studied hatha yoga. He is a great authority on the subject of yoga. Behind him are over 45 years of daily personal yoga practices. He is well acquainted with Vedanta, Samkhya philosophy, and the Sanskrit language. He is also a master in Indian classical music as well as a classical piano player.

Yogi Darshan is a practical yogi, a man of great mystical sensibility. He has dedicated his entire life to the practice of meditation and to the loving services of humankind. He spent many years meditating in isolated places in deep forests of the mysterious Himalayas, surrounded by great realized masters, in order to obtain personal experiences. He has many spiritual devotees in India. He also has trained hundreds of yoga teachers in France and in the United States. He has inspired and awakened several sincere yoga seekers into the esoteric transcendental yoga.

He said that he has waited to arrive at the peak of his yoga experiences before writing this book. It is the product of his over 45 years of daily practice of holistic yoga. There are already many books written on the subject of yoga, but this one is unique, as it offers the experiences and the thoughts of a living master to arrive at a Self-discovery.

www.ingramcontent.com/pod-product-compliance
Lightning Source LLC
Chambersburg PA
CBHW032135020426
42334CB00016B/1172